American Medical Association

Physicians dedicated to the health of America

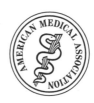

Assessing and Improving
Billing and Collections

D1609216

Prepared for
The American Medical Association
Cam McClellan Teems
The Coker Group

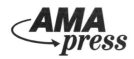

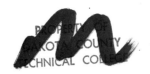

Assessing and Improving Billing and Collections

Internet address: www.ama-assn.org

This book is for informational purposes only. It is not intended to constitute legal or financial advice. If legal, financial, or other professional advice is required, the services of a competent professional should be sought.

Additional copies of this book may be ordered by calling 800-621-8335. Secure on-line orders can be taken at www.ama-assn.org/catalog. Mention product number OP318600.

ISBN 1-57947-078-5
BP38:0093-00:9/00

THE COKER GROUP is a national provider of health care consultative and management services assisting physicians, hospitals, and health care systems to better position themselves to be successful in a reformed health care environment. THE COKER GROUP offers a broad spectrum of programs and services for its clients.

- Primary Care Physician Network Development
- Practice Valuations and Acquisition Negotiations
- Physician Employment and Compensation Contract Design
- Facilitation of Group Practice Development
- Physician Practice Management Services
- Management Services Organization (MSO) Development
- Market Share Management Program
- Newly Recruited Physician Services
- Educational Programs
- Evaluation and Consultant Services
- Personnel Productivity Programs
- *PRACTICE SUCCESS!*© and *PRACTICE SUCCESS!*© Series

For more information, contact

> The Coker Group
> 11660 Alpharetta Highway
> Building 700, Ste 710
> Roswell, GA 30076
> 678 832-2000
> www.cokergroup.com

ABOUT THE AUTHOR

Cam McClellan Teems holds the position of Principal with The Coker Group, a national health care consulting firm based in Atlanta, Georgia. Prior to joining The Coker Group, Ms Teems served as a corporate officer of a major orthopaedic group practice with multiple state locations. During her tenure with the specialty group, she also served as the director of marketing and business development, where she implemented over $5 million in ancillary revenue sources and patient retention programs.

After receiving her undergraduate and graduate degrees from the University of Georgia (Athens), Ms Teems continued her focus on business communication and strategy, serving as an adjunct professor at the University of North Florida (Jacksonville). In this position, she taught a varied curriculum at the School of Business and Department of Communications. Later, she served as marketing and business development director for a Fortune 1000 company in the Southeast and a large computer manufacturer in the northeastern United States.

Cam Teems' background and areas of concentration include marketing and business development; ancillary revenue identification and implementation; market research and analysis; strategic planning and market forecasting; and customer retention planning and program implementation. In her position with The Coker Group, Ms Teems offers practice management consulting along with seasoned strategic planning to help clients meet current and future demands. She is a member of the editorial advisory board for *Practice Marketing and Management* newsletter and a candidate for fellowship in the American College of Medical Practice Executives of the Medical Group Management Association.

ssessing and Improving Billing and Collections is one of a series of books written to provide assessment tools and systematic processes to enable internal examination of the strengths and weaknesses of business operations. Decreasing reimbursement requires practices to be as operationally perceptive as possible. If your practice is feeling a financial pinch, you need to know why. But knowing where and how to look for information can be overwhelming without a plan and a process.

The purpose of this book is to provide a systematic approach to reviewing the billing office. It is a guide to assessment that makes possible the determination of what is and is not working. It recommends systems and policies that will work better in today's marketplace. It provides background information to help practices that elect to engage outside assistance in developing and implementing new procedures to be better prepared to participate and move forward. Included with this book is a diskette that contains many of the sample tables and forms in Microsoft Word® 6.0 for you to adapt, personalize, and modify for you and your practice.

This book and the others in the *Assessing and Improving Practice Operations©* Series are intended to offer concrete, practical information on topics sometimes considered the least important aspect of the profession of medicine: the business of running a medical practice. The long, hard years you dedicated to medical school and residency training were meant to make you an excellent physician, not an excellent businessperson. Caring for patients is and always will be your first priority. However, you cannot successfully run a medical practice without planning and without consideration of important business issues. While it takes a minimum of 10 years to become a physician, the day a practice opens is the day a physician becomes a small businessperson.

Your education probably did not include much information on medical office operations, personnel management, accounting, or business law. Yet, these business issues are more important than ever before, because the practice of medicine is far more complex than ever before. Good business management is essential to good medical practice. The physician who ignores basic business principles may soon face difficulties with suppliers, employees, the government, or patients.

Other pressures contribute to the need to seek greater efficiency. Most physicians find demands on their time increasing exponentially. There is a daily struggle to build a practice that will earn a steady income, to schedule regular working hours, to deliver quality care to patients, and to still have

PREFACE

time for relaxation and family. Developing an efficient practice makes all of these attainable. The application of good business planning will enable you to spend more time on the things that are most important to you.

This book and the others in the *Assessing and Improving Practice Operations*© series are guides to medical practice management for both the new physician and the established physician. They are not intended to provide solutions to every challenge that may arise. Their goal is to acquaint you with essential business principles and tools, as well as with some new approaches to managing your practice. The information they provide can be supplemented with information you gather from your colleagues and advisors. You will then be in a position to explore those ideas that promise to achieve the best results for your particular situation.

By providing the information in this book and others, the American Medical Association (AMA) is not endorsing any one management philosophy or method of delivering health care services. No single approach will meet the objectives of all physicians. Physicians and their staffs have to decide for themselves the best way to manage their individual practices. Finally, this book does not enunciate AMA policy. The annual *Policy Compendium* of the AMA sets forth our positions on such issues as contracting, medical ethics, managed care, and practice management.

We hope that this publication will be useful to you.

The American Medical Association

The systematic process in this book is a chronicle of an actual assessment of the billing and collections function of Associates in Orthopaedics and Sports Medicine, PC, of Dalton, Georgia. The physicians in this practice found themselves working harder, staying busier, and yet collecting far less than they were entitled to receive for the level of services they were performing. They were preparing to add another physician to their group of three, which forced them to take a hard look at where they were financially—and to ask whether they should be doing better.

Associates in Orthopaedics and Sports Medicine engaged The Coker Group to analyze billing and collections procedures and to recommend remedies for improving the processes. The practice had simply outgrown its billing and collections systems. Steps that had worked prior to the growth of managed care were no longer effective. This book grew out of the experience at Orthopaedics and Sports Medicine, and the author expresses much appreciation to them.

The purpose of this book is to help key members of a medical practice self-assess their billing and collections policies and procedures to discover problems and prevent undue financial losses. To the physicians who let us step in and look at their problems, we say thank you. Because of your graciousness, other physicians will be more able to make effective changes that ultimately will help the public at large.

CONTENTS

INDEX. LIST OF FIGURES, FORMS, AND TABLES

CHAPTER 1

Getting Ready for a Self-Assessment

The purpose of this book is to present a method of assessment that, when used continually or periodically, will improve practice operations. In the typical practice, staff members follow the work routines taught them by their managers or their predecessors. Staff members also have developed methods that make sense to them. Some—in fact, many—of these systems work well. Others, however, have become outdated as a result of changes in billing and collections forced on medical practices by the marketplace. The hurried pace of the practice environment often keeps staff members or managers from being able to augment their procedures—even if they know they are flawed.

Because previous routines may no longer be as effective as they were in the past, every practice should assess its billing and collections department to gain insight into the state of affairs. Although it may be preferable to engage an outside reviewer to maintain objectivity, doing so is not necessary. This chapter will help physicians and practice managers pull together the information to assess the results and then to analyze the methods in place.

GATHERING YOUR DATA

To begin the billing and collections assessment, you will need to review a number of important documents. The first step, therefore, is to gather key practice data and to have it on hand for the steps that will follow. **Table 1-1** is a billings and collections assessment checklist to use to begin gathering this data.

Whether the billing and collections assessment was initiated by the physician-owners of a practice, by the employer, such as a health system

TABLE 1-1. BILLING AND COLLECTIONS ASSESSMENT CHECKLIST

Collect the following documents before starting the assessment.

_____ **1.** Physician CVs

_____ **2.** Sample charge master (or superbill)

_____ **3.** Sample hospital billing information sheet or billing card (used to document hospital procedures performed during emergency room call and scheduled surgical procedures)

_____ **4.** Accounts receivable aging report for the practice (preferably 0–180 + days)

_____ **5.** Accounts receivable by physician

_____ **6.** Accounts receivable by payer

_____ **7.** Accounts receivable by location (eg, satellite offices)

_____ **8.** Collections report documenting gross charges versus net collections and corresponding adjustment rates—by month of current period and previous fiscal year-to-date

_____ **9.** Income statement for the most recent period and previous fiscal year-to-date

_____ **10.** Procedure report by month for the most recent period and previous fiscal year-to-date (by top 50 codes)

_____ **11.** Procedure report (CPT codes) by month by physician

_____ **12.** Procedure report (CBP codes) by monthly by facility

_____ **13.** Tax return for prior calendar year

_____ **14.** Listing of referral sources and corresponding referral numbers, by month, for most recent period

_____ **15.** Sample practice collection letters, if any

_____ **16.** List of hospital participation and corresponding privilege levels

_____ **17.** List of participating payers

_____ **18.** Sample of 25 explanations of benefits (EOBs) and 5 remittance advice forms (mixture of clean and unclean claims)

_____ **19.** Sample error report from electronic claims filing procedure

_____ **20.** Sample statement for patient responsible balances

_____ **21.** Description of practice management and billing software system and capabilities

_____ **22.** List of staff members, job descriptions, and salaries

_____ **23.** Samples of all internal reports currently generated by the practice for billing and collections review

_____ **24.** Patient demographic data by age and by zip code

_____ **25.** Copies of all managed care contracts

_____ **26.** Copy of practice fee schedule listing all codes

_____ **27.** Sample patient information sheet

Note: _If the financial statements contain codes, abbreviations, or other information not easily identifiable, it is wise to have a key available that outlines the corresponding meanings of those codes or abbreviations (eg, MC = Medicare, MD = Medicaid, Physician Code 013 = Dr Smith). Keep this list nearby during the review process._

that owns the practice and employs the physicians, or by employed physicians, it is important to involve the physicians in the process and it is essential to have their cooperation and support. Interviews with physicians are one of the foundational steps in the progression.

Interview the physicians with the expectations of uncovering their specific concerns. Make it possible for them to be introspective and open. For example, a physician may tell you that he or she is busier than ever—seeing more patients, performing more procedures—yet the cash flow may be surprisingly sparse. Or perhaps a physician has noticed unusual behavior on the part of another staff member that he or she previously has been reluctant to discuss.

Explain the process. Set expectations for the assessment and a time line for completion of the process. It is important to set deadlines and meet them. Go through the checklist of information with the physicians, and explain each document on the list and how it will be used in the assessment.

UNDERSTANDING YOUR PRACTICE INFORMATION

The documents you gather will provide the information you need to assess the practice. Ensure that all the documents are together before getting started.

Begin by reviewing the income statement. Often an income statement will point out obvious areas of trouble, such as expenses that are higher than the norm or a revenue shortfall.

Next, review the accounts receivable aging report. Keeping this report up to date is an integral part of the billing and collections manager's daily routine. The report should show the practice's success in collections by payer. Some obvious areas to look at are the percentage of receivables by aging category and the total receivables. Ideally, there should be no more than 4 months of operating expense in the receivables, and no more than 20% of the entire amount should be more than 90 days old.

After reviewing the accounts receivable aging report, look over the report that shows the adjustment rate (ie, gross charges versus net charges). Several sources provide information on acceptable adjustment rates by specialty, such as Medical Group Management Association (MGMA) and American Medical Group Association (AMGA). Generally, adjustments to billed charges should not total more than 40%.

Finally, review the collections adjustments. Using benchmarks obtained from sources such as the aforementioned and specialty academies, look at the performance standards of other practices. These benchmark reports are usually available from these sources at a significant cost. However, associations that provide such material often offer discounts on the purchase to their members. Although these items come at an expense, they are often worthwhile sources as comparables. The specialty academies are beginning to gather this sort of data in the future and will be able to offer it by specialty, as opposed to a volume that addresses appropriate billing and collections levels for all specialties across all regions of the United States.

Create a chart and mark your position on the chart. Does your practice fall in the 25%, 50%, or 75% range? Typically, you will want to rank in the 50th percentile at a minimum in a heavily managed care market, and at least in the 75th percentile in a low managed care environment.

The objective in this initial exercise is to review the documents from a fresh perspective. Later, we will examine each item for the purpose of completing the assessment.

MAKING A CURSORY REVIEW

Use the billings and assessment checklist and the review of practice information to make a note of each obvious problem and to develop a list of questions. Include the areas that you think may contribute to potential collections problems. Often, your instincts are right. Plan to go back to these questions later, and record your assumptions as answers become available. Once you have created this list, use it to create an action plan for addressing the problem areas.

FOLLOWING THE PATIENT ENCOUNTER

Review each step of the patient encounter—starting when a patient calls in for an appointment. Write down what the telephone attendant tells the patient and what information is obtained from the patient. Then ask yourself the following questions:

- Is complete and accurate demographic information entered into the computer as the call is made?
- Does the telephone attendant schedule the appointment?
- Does the attendant tell the patient about billing policies and collection procedures?
- Will the patient arrive at the practice on the day and time of the appointment prepared to pay for the services rendered using cash, a check, or a credit card, or by submitting an insurance claim?

- Is a brochure describing the practice, the hours of operation, the physician profiles, and billing policies mailed to the patient?
- Is the patient asked to complete a patient information sheet with all relevant guarantor, employer, and demographic information while he or she is at the office?
- How does the front office verify eligibility of coverage for patients with a third-party payer?

Details about copayments, deductibles, and noncovered services can be gathered when the patient presents for the encounter and verified while the physician is examining the patient. With the proper demographic profile, it is easier to collect the appropriate payment for noncovered items before the patient leaves the office.

Often, money is lost on the front end of the patient encounter because staff members are hesitant about obtaining the proper level of information. In Chapter 2, we will advise on key points in the office encounter that will result in better collections. The initial step, however, is to monitor the process and comment on the details as they arise.

CONCLUSION

The initial planning of an assessment of the practices' billing and collections process is often the most crucial stage. Gather all relevant materials together and review them. Make notes as you follow the collection process through the entire patient encounter. This is an excellent opportunity to observe a process that may have become invisible to the day-to-day manager or physician.

CHAPTER 2

Tracking the Patient Encounter

A patient encounter begins with the first call to the practice by a prospective patient. The collection process also begins at the first call, and that is when the success or failure of the collection process is set up. The dialogue that occurs between the patient and the telephone attendant or receptionist during the first episode determines whether the patient will be cooperative about making sure that the physician is compensated for his or her time.

CONDUCTING FRONT OFFICE STAFF INTERVIEWS

Staff interviews can often reveal mistakes that potentially become obstacles to collection. The interview process can also reveal strengths and weaknesses that can later be adjusted to improve the billing and collections process. Often, the staff members who are in daily contact with patients and processes have the most information about how to improve the processes. It is advisable to query staff members at least quarterly to find out their ideas on process improvement, not just for billing and collections but for all practice management processes.

Practice Manager

Quite possibly, the practice administrator or manager is conducting the review of the billing office. Nevertheless, all functions need to be examined for efficiencies—even if this entails self-examination.

The practice manager should relate the steps that occur in the office encounter, and these steps should be recorded in writing. Putting procedures on paper is one way of seeing where there are loopholes and where improvements can be made to benefit business operations. Begin by chronicling the encounter from start to finish—from the time the patient contacts the practice by telephone to set up an appointment, all the way through the completion of the medical record and the resolution of any outstanding accounts receivable.

Receptionist

The receptionist or the staff member who answers the telephone to make patient appointments is often the first person who discusses anything to do with the practice, the patient, and the financial relationship between the two. Ensure that the receptionist is well aware of all the financial parameters established by the practice.

Let us start with the person who answers the telephone and schedules the appointments. Typically, this staff member's role is to listen to the patient's request for a time slot that is convenient and to match that time with available slots on the appointment schedule. Although this is the most important first step in any patient encounter, it is only the first step in setting up an accurate patient process.

Once the appointment is scheduled, it is important to collect information that will make it easier for the patient to participate in the practice's billing and collection process. Often, if this part of the process is not completed, the rest of the process suffers. We recommend using the initial telephone call to gather information about the patient's insurance or managed care plan, copayments and/or deductibles, and guarantor information. These particulars then can be verified before the patient arrives for the appointment. When accurate enrollment data is housed in the practice, the patient can be matched to the enrollment data, and coverage can be verified. In addition, coverage has already been verified when the patient arrives at the practice, speeding up the process of checking in the patient. If there is an information sheet upon arrival at the medical practice, each new patient should complete it. This should provide information about the patient's address, employer, primary and secondary insurance, subscriber, etc. Each patient should be asked when registering with the office if his or her address has changed on any of the insurance information.

Billing Clerk

The billing clerk is usually responsible for handling the patient's financial information once the encounter has culminated, the copayment or deductible has been collected, and the patient has left the premises. Usually, the billing clerk sees the patient encounter information and verifies the information on it. For example, the billing clerk checks for accurate coding—ie, *Current Procedural Technology™ (CPT) 2000*[1] and *The*

International Classification of Diseases, 9th Revision, Clinical Modification (ICD-9)[2]—that will result in a clean claim. Traditionally, a *clean* claim is a claim that is processed without incident and paid appropriately based on a managed care contracted rate of reimbursement or other standard payment arrangement. An *unclean* claim results in an EOB that rejects all or part of the itemized billing of an encounter and documents this rejection with applicable reason codes. Additionally, the billing clerk will also ensure that the claim is sent to the payer in a timely fashion after the encounter. *Timely* should mean between 24 and 48 hours after the date of service.

Traditionally, an insurance specialist participates in the billing and collections process once a claim has been sent to the payer for payment and either a payment has been received or there is correspondence about the claim. Depending on the size of the practice, insurance specialists typically are organized by payer, and they follow up on claims submitted to the payers they are responsible for. For example, an insurance specialist assigned to Medicare follows up on all outstanding claims for Medicare patients and handles correspondence requiring further medical record information or information about the encounter.

Insurance Specialist

CONCLUSION

Every staff member has a responsibility toward the patient and the patient's participation in the billing and collections process. It is often helpful to periodically interview each staff member to ascertain whether changes to the billing and collections process should be made, based on patient demographic changes, managed care participation changes, provider changes within the practice, or any other augmentations to the practice management function.

Interviewing staff members is often the best way to reveal problems in the billing and collections process. If you can constantly improve the efficiency of this flow of information, you can often preclude an increase in outstanding accounts receivable.

Endnotes

1. American Medical Association. *Current Procedural Technology*™ *(CPT) 2000*. Chicago, Ill: American Medical Association; 1999.

2. Medicode, Inc. *The International Classification of Diseases, 9th Revision, Clinical Modification (ICD-9)*. Salt Lake City, Utah: Ingenix Publishing; 1998.

CHAPTER 3

Completing the Analysis

Use the data you collected in Table 1-1 to obtain an overview of the practice's billing and collections. Note your observations, and make recommendations for improvement in each of the categories discussed in this chapter: accounts receivable; collection levels; departmental administrative direction and leadership; operational organization; computer systems and technological processes; department personnel training; policy and procedures manual; adjustment process; copayment collection; staffing levels; management reports; charge capture; compliance plan; internal controls and cash handling; coding; managed care information; and physical facility. In the end, the conclusions that will come from the analysis will form the plan for improving the billing and collections department.

ACCOUNTS RECEIVABLE

In Chapter 1 we describe the benefits of benchmark usage as a way to compare or assess your billing and collections process. Using benchmarks obtained from the MGMA, AMGA, or the appropriate specialty society, plot your practice's accounts receivables against national norms for your specialty. Ask the following questions:

- Are the levels greater than normal? If so, what is the variance?
- Where are the balances in the aging categories? Account balances that are at or above 180 days are difficult to collect.
- What classifications of balances are in the past-due categories? Accounts classified as *self-pay* are particularly difficult to collect. Self-pay accounts are patients who are either uninsured or who are covered by insurance plans that the practice does not participate in. Also, some balances are the patient's responsibility after insurance claims have been paid.

Some remedies can help with the typical problems that an accounts receivable analysis reveals. To begin, hire an experienced, energetic, well-organized central business office manager to assume responsibility for all daily operations. The office manager should have specific, realistic, and attainable accounts receivable target goals and should have the authority to make staffing changes to improve efficiency and increase collections in order to reduce accounts receivable levels.

Devise a management reporting system that provides basic information about cash collections and accounts receivable levels. The reports should be run frequently and should compare actual results to predetermined targets. They should be given to the physicians on a monthly basis to review. Also, update the billing and collections computer software to improve efficiency of claims processing and collection activities.

Create a task force of experienced collection personnel to reduce accounts receivable levels. Beginning with the 90-day category, work all accounts of any amount. Then work only the larger accounts in the older aging categories (ie, more than 90 days past due). Give task force members an incentive to achieve above-average collection results. Avoid turning these balances over to a collection agency at this juncture.

COLLECTION LEVELS

What is the practice's gross collection percentage? How does this number compare to a normal gross collection percentage for a practice in its specialty? As indicated earlier, benchmarks for these comparisons can be obtained through MGMA, AMGA, and specialty society organizations.

If the percentages are too high in comparison to other practices, the collection process is probably flawed. If this is the case, interview the insurance specialist in the practice to get answers to these questions:

- What is the policy for account follow-up?
- How often are patient statements sent?
- Does the statement post adjustments for payments made by insurance payers? Does it identify who makes the payments or who is expected to make payment?
- Can statement messages be predetermined, customized, or selectively withheld?

If collection levels are too low based on gross collection percentages, begin by streamlining the insurance specialist's routines to reduce the volume of nonaccount follow-up activities. Establish a collections group with the primary responsibility for collecting all patient-responsible balances aged more than 60 days. Collection of all insurance accounts should remain with the insurance specialist regardless of account aging. The collections group could form the basis of a regular function within the billing and collections department.

Modify the standard statement so that it is used only when the entire balance due is the patient's responsibility. For cases when insurance copayments, deductibles, or noncovered balances are involved, generate a specific patient statement, withholding the standard messages and adding customized collection messages to correspond with the account status. Also, print outstanding balances on the encounter form to alert the provider and other staff members to route the patient for financial counseling before leaving the practice.

DEPARTMENTAL ADMINISTRATIVE DIRECTION AND LEADERSHIP

Effective management and leadership is key to a successful billing and collections department. The manager must function as a leader and a motivator. The manager should be aware of the status of the accounts receivable, days in accounts receivable, and collection percentage for the area of responsibility. He or she should monitor all activity that goes on in the department, use motivational techniques and incentives, and keep an eye on workloads and accomplishments of the staff. The accounts receivable manager should be regarded as a knowledgeable resource in billing and collections methods. The manager should also be known for giving credit to others and acknowledging their value.

The accounts receivable manager, who is responsible for all daily operations, should have specific attainable accounts receivable goals. This manager should have the authority to make staffing changes that will improve departmental efficiency in increasing collections and reducing accounts receivables.

By recognizing staff members for a job well done when goals are achieved, the accounts receivable manager inspires staff members by providing recognition for maintaining heavy workloads, accomplishing above average collections, or reducing accounts receivable levels. Each staff member should have a measurable, reasonable, and attainable goal and should receive recognition and rewards for attaining or exceeding that goal. The incentives can be monetary or promotional, such as gift certificates, coffee mugs, or practice-specific certificates of achievement. The accounts receivable manager should institute an incentive plan for all members of the department to encourage them to exceed goals. Also, if the front office staff has an incentive as well, they will be sure to get correct insurance information up front and to check eligibility. The manager should also receive an incentive that is a significant component of his or her compensation plan.

OPERATIONAL ORGANIZATION

Problems and inefficiencies often result from assigning too many functions to a single staff member. For example, if an insurance specialist is responsible for a specified physician's billing and collection from claims generation through both insurance and patient-responsible balance follow-up, it is unlikely that sufficient time will be available for daily routine billing functions in addition to collection functions.

Typically, insurance specialists do not have time to work the accounts receivable list for collections. When time is available, most focus on the 180-day category. The 180-day category is the least likely to be collected, however. As a result, the greatest amount of time is spent on efforts that will be the least productive.

To improve operational organization, instruct insurance specialists to work insurance accounts in all aged categories. Remove mundane processing tasks, such as reviewing the daily patient visit list. Institute electronic claims filing to reduce the volume of claims that must be manually scanned to verify completeness. Electronic claims filing also eliminates the need for the insurance specialist to fold the claim, stuff the envelope, and mail the claim to the insurance company—manual tasks that are routine, clerical in nature, and do not require specialized knowledge.

COMPUTER SYSTEMS AND TECHNOLOGICAL PROCESSES

A look at the billing and collection process will show whether the process is labor-intensive or automated. Note the following:

- Is the process well organized?
- Does the process require manual intervention to ensure continued processing information?
- How much time is being spent on manual applications, such as copying checks?
- To what degree are claims being filed electronically?
- How well does the information system function? Is it reliable, or is it prone to lock up?
- How functional are the screen fields for capturing information?
- What tools are being used? Electronic claims filing for all payers? Scanning technology for encounter form input? Electronic remittance posting for Medicare? Use of a lock-box service through a financial institution? Other?

- What plans are in the works for upgrading the electronic billing and collections system?

Upgrade the computer system and technological processes to improve billing and collections functions. An upgraded computer system should include a powerful, effective, and reliable practice management and billing and collections program. Establishing electronic claims filing for as many payers as possible, including Medicare, will save staff members a considerable amount of time. Use a commercial clearinghouse service for claims that cannot be submitted directly to the payer. Contract for a lock-box service with a bank if the volume of payment warrants it. The bank will receive payments, copy the checks, deposit them to the proper account, and send deposit information daily. Ensure that the volume of payments is such that it would be a cost-sharing measure to implement such a service. Most lock-box services are costly. Make an all-out effort to catch up on posting explanations of benefits (EOB), even if doing so requires hiring temporary employees for data input.

DEPARTMENT PERSONNEL TRAINING

When computer hardware and/or software are replaced, it is necessary to train staff members to use the new program or technology. Conduct the training away from the office if possible so staff members can concentrate on learning the new software. Otherwise, the staff members may be continually pulled out of or interrupted during the training. Training includes teaching staff members how to capture demographic and insurance data for consistency in submitting clean insurance claims. It also includes cross-training.

Training should begin with an initial training cycle for all personnel. Two months later, hold a follow-up training session. Include all staff members, including those working in satellite offices and business sites for the practice. Provide additional training to staff members who have high input error rates, with special attention to checking or proofing for errors. Adjust staffing assignments and work flow to accomplish accurate and timely data input. Establish and reinforce performance parameters and goals with positive financial incentives.

POLICIES AND PROCEDURES MANUAL

A policies and procedures manual is essential to the smooth operation of any medical practice, particularly in its billing office. Without written policies, the billing and collections department is certain to be plagued with inconsistencies and questionable processes. The questions to ask about a policy and procedures manual are as follows:

- Is a written manual of policies and procedures in place?
- Who is responsible for keeping the manual up to date?
- How often are the policies updated?
- Who is responsible for enforcing the policies once they are in place?

Develop a billing and collections policy and procedures manual in concert with the implementation of new management software. The manual should include instructions on every function. It should cover special situations, such as reinstatement of adjustments when payments are received from secondary payers, reversal of write-offs, refund processes, application of credit balances to prior or subsequent patients visits, and so on. It should require periodic management reports, including those used to monitor departmental performance. Develop a financial policy to mail to patients before the first visit or hand to them when they come into the office for the encounter.

Enforcement of policies and procedures necessarily follows establishment. What good is it to have a credit policy, for example, that is ignored or disregarded?

ADJUSTMENT PROCESS

Adjusting charges for contractually discounted payments is an important step in the billing and collections function. The adjustment process is significant for the practice's success and viability. To be effective, routines must be simple.

Contract adjustment routines, corrections to patient accounts, and charge or posting error reversals should not be confused with other types of adjustments, such as refund requests, bad debt write-offs, collection referrals, and professional courtesies. It is important to differentiate the types of balances that require approval. Refunds, contractual adjustments, and bad debt and collection adjustment processes should be separate and distinct.

To be able to judge the appropriateness of payments and adjustments, staff members must know the contracted amounts for various payers under managed care agreements. This will ensure that insurance-generated EOBs are accurate in relation to the contracted fees. Staff members who post payments to accounts should use a matrix listing the contracted fees for the most common CPT™ codes so that reimbursements can be compared to the contracted amounts.

Approvals for contractual adjustments should be made by the billing and collections manager responsible for the collection ratio and accounts receivable levels. The practice manager and the physicians should monitor the adjustment procedures monthly.

COPAYMENT COLLECTION

Copayments (copays) represent significant revenue to the medical practice and should be regarded as a mandatory part of the patient encounter. A typical practice generates $5,000 to $10,000 in revenue from copays per physician per year. Failure to collect the copay from the patient is a violation of the typical managed care contract.

Most patients are expected to make payments—either copays or patient-responsible portions of estimated charges—during the encounter. Each patient should be asked to pay past-due balances or to arrange a payment plan for paying off the balances.

A billing and collections assessment should include the following questions:

- If the patient's insurance coverage includes a copay, is he or she asked to make the payment when presenting for the encounter?
- For patients in indemnity plans, is collecting patient-responsible portions routine at checkout?

Recommendations for improvement in cash flow and reduction of accounts receivable require asking for money at the time of service. Collect copayments at check-in. Patients expect to make this payment, which can be paid by cash, check, or credit card. Institute a procedure for collecting past-due balances at checkout. This may involve flagging the charge ticket with a special sticker or creating a place on the charge ticket area for indication of past-due balances. Request for payment should be handled privately by an experienced collections specialist.

Although many patients will prefer to pay patient-responsible balances after the physician receives the insurance payment, it is reasonable to ask for payment when deductibles have not been met. For example, it is reasonable to assume that deductibles have not been met in the early part of a year.

STAFFING LEVELS

Achieving appropriate billing and collections staffing is difficult at best. Assessment includes review of workload, processes, and automation.

Consider the following:

- How many full-time employees or full-time equivalents are assigned to the billing and collections department?
- What are the benchmarks for staffing according to MGMA, AMGA, and specialty society data?
- Are staff members keeping up with their workload, or are they asked to work overtime on a regular basis? Are they currently behind on their tasks?
- What expectations are set for billing and collections ratios, if any?
- What incentives, if any, are in place to promote objectives?

If the department is not keeping up with its tasks and is behind in the billing and collections process, engage a temporary employee to assist or ask a staff member from a different area to help out. This may entail after-hours work on weekends or evenings. Review procedures to eliminate unnecessary steps and inefficiencies. Offer incentives for meeting billing and collection goals to reduce past-due accounts receivable and improve collection rates.

MANAGEMENT REPORTS

Management reports are vital to the practice's lifeblood—its revenue stream and cash flow. Such crucial management reports as aged insurance claims pending, open claims, and insurance-specific aged receivables help management assess the position and manage billings and collections. Access to and use of data is another area for assessment. Following are questions to consider:

- What reports are currently being generated, how often are they run, and how are they used?
- What other reports are available through the information system? How would they help improve the billing and collections process?

Determine reporting requirements. Some examples of helpful reports are activity count, amount billed and collected, accounts receivable, and collection ratios. Ensure that the proper level of software technology is available for the practice. Ensure that the billing and collections department manager is capable of training staff members on report writing features and report analysis.

CHARGE CAPTURE

Reviewing the charge capture procedures is another fundamental area of billing and collections assessment. A great deal of revenue can be lost if patient encounters take place and procedures are performed that are not listed on encounter forms, and if the information from the forms (such as laboratory testing) does not make it to the billing system. An assessment should include the following questions:

- What is the control system for encounter forms? Are they prenumbered, automatically numbered, or not numbered?
- What are the processes for capturing surgery charges?
- Is a cross-check system in place?

Institute an automatic encounter form control system, such as prenumbering or automated numbering. Implement an audit control to ensure that all encounter forms are submitted daily. This can be done by comparing the patient sign-in log with the numbered encounter forms. Implement a charge capture audit process at the CPT™ service level. Implement a cross-check of hospital and surgery charge capture by comparing outside source documents with internal billing documents. Conduct periodic random audits to ensure that all charges are captured and billed.

COMPLIANCE PLAN

Having a compliance plan is strongly encouraged to avoid being charged with Medicare fraud and abuse. Although not yet required by law, having an established compliance plan in place is a good defensive strategy. An assessment should include the following questions:

- Is a plan in place to ensure against Medicare fraud and abuse?
- If so, what does the plan entail?
- What level of training do physicians and staff members receive about compliance issues and the vulnerability of the practice?

Every practice should develop and circulate a plan and train staff members about compliance. Every member of the staff should know the penalties for Medicare fraud and abuse.

If preliminary or existing documents are in place, review and update them for presentation to senior management and physicians. Once final or revised documents are approved, implement and integrate the plan into the daily operations and into the policies and procedures of the billing and collections department. Conduct an annual training refresher program, and annually review compliance with antifraud statutes. Consider engaging an outside consultant to assist in the completion and review of the compliance plan.

INTERNAL CONTROLS AND CASH HANDLING

Setting up internal controls for handling payments and cash is mandatory for a medical practice. There are many opportunities for payments to disappear unless controls are in place that limit the likelihood of theft. Part of a billing and collections assessment must focus on the way payments are handled. Some of the important questions to ask about operation and management of incoming cash and payments concern how and when deposits are made, posted, and recorded.

Deposit checks and cash payments daily, unless the amounts are so small they do not warrant the effort. Prepare a deposit slip every day, and show a total for that day. If you skip a day, make two deposits the next day. This verifies that all funds received on a given day were deposited. Record each receivable separately on the deposit slip. This provides a good audit trail and serves as proper documentation for posting the receivable. Posting reports back up the deposit slip.

Copy each insurance check, and attach the copy to the explanation of benefits. Copy each patient check and attach it to a Daily Collections Summary Worksheet. See **Table 3-1** for a sample worksheet. Enter the check number for bulk checks. This allows a particular check to match the EOB that comes with it. It also provides a way to track payments, if needed.

TABLE 3-1. SAMPLE DAILY COLLECTIONS SUMMARY SHEET

ABC Practice Daily Collections Summary Sheet					
Date	Patient Acct #	Last Name	Check #	Payer	Total Amount Received
10-12-00	123456	Smith	2345	Self	$ 255.00
10-12-00	123457	Jones	222	Cigna	$1200.34
10-12-00	123458	Brown	1427	Cigna	$ 556.02

Cash paid to physicians, such as honoraria, rental income, interest income, and other fees for nonmedical services, should not be included in the practice deposits. Maintain a log to track these payments as they are received. Give the physicians a copy and retain another in the accounting department for record-keeping purposes. Any income not related to patients' fees (eg, fees for making copies of medical records) should be deposited into the practice's operating account and must be posted to the daily journal to reconcile charges and receipts and to prevent overstatement of the collection rate at month end and year end.

Manage cash flow on a daily basis. Use a basic summary sheet to track cash flow as follows:

$$\begin{array}{c} Beginning \\ balance \end{array} + \begin{array}{c} Current\ day \\ deposits \end{array} - \begin{array}{c} Current\ day \\ disbursements \end{array} = \begin{array}{c} Ending \\ balance \end{array}$$

Reconcile the bank statement and financial statement book balance each month to be certain of an accurate cash flow. Look at trends to anticipate cash inflow and outflow. Disbursements and reimbursements should be predictable. Unexpected changes should be a signal that investigation is needed.

A system of internal checks and balances helps preclude innocent errors and deliberate fraud. The key is to separate handling of cash from the accounting records. One staff member receives the cash; another posts it to the books; and a third deposits it in the checking account.

Another alternative—when the volume of checks warrants it—is to use the bank's lock-box service. Payments are mailed directly to the lock-box address and deposited as received. The bank then sends deposit amounts and copies of checks to the practice for posting to the patients' accounts. This increases security and provides an additional cross-check for payment posting. For example, a report should be run daily of total charges and total payments. A different person should run a calculator tape off of the charge tickets of charges and payments. Each report should be given to the practice manager who compares to see if the reports balance.

CODING

Procedural coding must be accurate. A billing and collections assessment should include an audit to ensure compliance and legitimate maximization of fees. The questions to ask are as follows:

- Who codes procedures?
- Who reviews the coding of procedures?
- By what means is coding information transmitted to the billing mechanism?
- Is insurance coverage verified in advance of procedures? Do problems occur as a result of precertification or lack of coverage?
- How are variations in the way payers want surgical procedures reported—separately or as part of the major procedure—tracked to avoid appeals and write-offs?

Conduct periodic audits of the complete coding process through a procedural coding analysis to ensure compliance and maximization of fees. Maintain detailed information on the peculiarities of each payer, and meet their specific requirements and variances to avoid inappropriate adjustments or the need for appeals.

MANAGED CARE INFORMATION

Practices frequently lose money because of a lack of information about the specifics of managed care contracts and the requirements of each plan. The billing and collections department must have current information for providers about each plan, the contracted fees for the most common CPT™ codes, and coverage and billing procedures for physician assistant services. An assessment should focus on the following questions:

- What information is at hand about each plan? How is it updated?
- Does the information include the name of a plan service representative for each plan?
- How are appeals handled?

Develop a binder for each health plan that includes the contracted fees for the most common CPT™ codes, coverage, and billing procedures. Maintain a list of problems with this plan to be discussed during renegotiation of the contract. Provide the receptionist and clinical staff at each practice location with a requirement matrix. Maintain updates about provider applications in process, and monitor them at least weekly, reporting results to the billing office and the physician.

PHYSICAL FACILITY

Working space for the billing and collections function is often limited by the physical facility. Noise levels are usually high. An assessment of the billing and collections department should include observations on space limitations and recommendations for improvements. Consider relocating the billing and collections function to another site. Distribute telephone headsets for conducting calls that require concentration. Use space efficiently for office equipment such as scanners, copiers, files, and so on.

CONCLUSION

Most assessments of the billing and collections functions of a medical practice will reveal both strengths and weaknesses in operations. Successful operations have effective leadership, systems, policies, processes, technology, and reporting. The observations and recommendations listed in the chapter are a foundation for improving the billing and collections department.

CHAPTER 4

Setting Up the Billing and Collections Operations

As part of the assessment process for billing and collections, the practice manager or other staff member who is doing the assessment should go through the exercise of setting up the billing and collections process as if it does not exist. Often, pretending that the process is not currently in place and taking the opportunity to start anew will allow fresh thinking. You may end up creating a billing and collections process that is very distinct from the one in place, or you may just change parts of the process.

IDENTIFYING ROLES AND ASSIGNING RESPONSIBILITIES

The first step in setting up the collections process is identifying the personnel who participate in it. These staff members most likely have other roles in practice management, but some parts of their job descriptions deal with billing and collections.

A useful way to begin is to create a flowchart showing how the patient moves through the practice and how information about that patient is retrieved. **Figure 4-1** is a flowchart describing one practice prior to assessment and change.

EMPLOYING THE RIGHT PEOPLE

The key to successful billing and collections is employing the right people. Finding personnel who have the correct skills is often the most difficult part of setting up an efficient process.

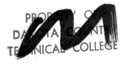

FIGURE 4-1. CURRENT SCENARIO FLOWCHART

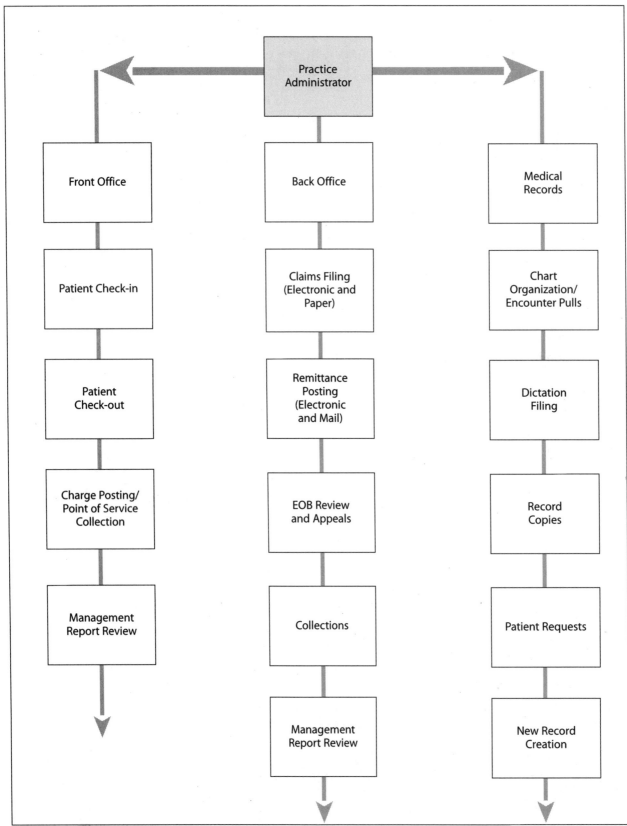

Start your assessment of the personnel who support the billing and collections process by making a list of all the staff members who participate in it. Remember to list staff members whose main responsibilities are not billing and collections but who have responsibilities related to the function, such as the practice's receptionist and switchboard operator.

When you have made the list, add the functions that staff members perform that support billing and collections data gathering and process improvement. Objectively assess whether those you have identified indeed have the right skills. For example, a traditional receptionist is crucial to the point of service (POS) collections process. Therefore, he or she must possess the following skill set:

- pleasant, yet direct communication style;
- ability to communicate to patients regarding their health care coverage;
- understanding of the necessity of all relevant demographic information gathering; and
- attentive to detail, such as accurate recording of social security or referral numbers.

Ask yourself whether each understands the value of his or her participation in the process. Most employees do not understand that they participate in a process and how important their one function is to the larger process. For example, a medical records clerk may assume that his or her task is simply one of filing. He or she may not understand how essential the documentation surrounding a patient's encounter is to the overall practice.

ESTABLISHING PAYMENT POLICIES AND FEES

A necessary part of assessing a billing and collections process is to determine whether there are policies and controls in place that efficiently garner payment information and actual payments from patients. The assessment also evaluates whether those payments are commensurate with the time and effort of providers and staff members who support the patient encounter.

If your practice does not have a billing and collections policy and procedures manual, we recommend that you create one. A manual will help you change the billing and collections processes. It also serves as excellent ongoing training and support for staff members when they have questions.

As consultants, we frequently encounter employees who tell us that policies are not in writing. They say that the practice manager has verbally communicated the policies and procedures. On further examination, we discover that each staff member who articulates the policies and procedures relates them quite differently. A written format helps ensure adherence to policies and averts inconsistencies in communication of the policies.

Identifying the correct charges or fees for professional services is often difficult. It does not have to be. Several associations publish fee data that can be compared to the fees being charged by your practice. In addition, data is available that supports recommended benchmarks for specialty fees by geographic regions of the United States. These data can help you compare your practice's fees with what other specialists or nonspecialists in your geographic region are charging.

Another way to evaluate your fees is to be aware of your practice's adjustment rate. The adjustment rate by specialty is also readily available to use as a comparison. If your practice's adjustment rate falls outside of the norm, this may indicate that the fees are inconsistent with the charging customs of similar providers in the market.

Physicians need to be aware of price-fixing issues. Physicians from different practices should not agree on what fees they will charge. However, a practice needs to evaluate its fees annually against published benchmarks to ensure that its prices are competitive.

USING PERFORMANCE STANDARDS FOR COLLECTORS

Using performance standards can help you determine how well insurance specialists and/or collectors are performing. These standards should be tied to the practice's monthly collection goals. Usually, the standards relate to the number of days it takes to collect outstanding balances and/or the collection rate of the practice by financial class.

REWARDING PERFORMANCE THROUGH BONUS PLANS

Often a practice will choose to reward its staff members for performance that contributes to increased collections and to a more pleasant patient experience. For example, a front office staff member might always greet patients with a smile, or an insurance specialist may have worked out a system for collecting a maximum amount for a special procedure.

Incentives can come in the form of certificates of recognition, gift certificates, promotional items, or cash bonuses. Other examples are

- a coffee cup with the name of the practice on the side,
- a T-shirt with the practice's logo,
- a gift certificate from a local bookstore,

- a gift certificate from a local restaurant,
- a free day off coupon that can be used for an additional paid vacation day,
- a plant for the employee's desk,
- a certificate to display on the wall or in the work area.

Remember, however, that these incentives and how these incentives are earned must be clearly defined.

APPLYING CODING KNOWLEDGE

Most billing and collections staff members need to have a cursory knowledge of coding, particularly the coding related to the specialty of the practice. A staff member who constantly has to refer to a CPT book is wasting valuable time.

Staff members should know the following basics about coding:

- Codes are added and deleted each year. They should be updated in the practice's information management system.
- Some codes traditionally stand alone and represent the entire procedure.
- Some codes are traditionally bundled with other codes to represent a procedure.
- Some codes require modifiers.
- All codes require documentation.
- Some codes, when incurred together, will be considered multiprocedural and be subject to a write-off.

CONCLUSION

During a billing and collections assessment, you have the opportunity to reset your billing and collections operations. This can range from the reevaluation of staff members and their skills to evaluation of the information management system used in the process. The assessment gives you a chance to step back and view the process from a fresh perspective.

CHAPTER 5

Getting Paid by the Patient

Payment from the patient is often the most overlooked area in the collection process. Because of the proliferation of managed care plans, it is easy to forget that not all of the cost will be reimbursed by a third party.

COLLECTING AT THE TIME OF SERVICE

While patients are in the office for treatment, verify their insurance information, and collect payments that are due. It is better to issue the patient a refund than to incur the cost of collecting an outstanding balance. A major goal should be to collect everything that is due when a patient comes to the office for an appointment. Of course, when payment by the patient is not allowed by law or contract, collecting does not apply. However, as many as 90% of patients have some form of payment responsibility at the time services are rendered.

The ability to collect appropriate funds begins with appointment scheduling protocol. The staff member who schedules appointments should know the practice's policies and should proactively express payment expectations at the time the appointment is scheduled. When questions arise, either during the scheduling process or when patients call in for information, the scheduler must be able to respond appropriately. Telling a new patient that all copayments and deductibles are due at the time of service is appropriate. This establishes the foundation for the collection policy at the outset of the relationship. The successful management of accounts receivable, billing, and collecting is a matter of establishing precedents and implementing policies consistently.

The receptionist should remind the patient about the payment policy when the patient presents for the encounter

> *Receptionist: It is our practice policy to collect appropriate monies due from the patient at the time service is rendered. This may be only your copay and deductible, but we do ask for payment at this time.*

Having the scheduler and the receptionist state the practice's payment policy will eliminate surprise and embarrassment when the request for payment is made at check-out.

The next step is the use of an encounter form (or superbill) for all office procedures. Routing well-designed forms to the staff member completing the check-out process allows for a smooth and efficient payment process. The charge information for the day's services will be easy to calculate and available when the patient is checking out. Depending on the practice's policy, the staff member completing the check-out process can make a statement similar to any of the following.

> *Staff member: Your charges for today's visit are $50, Mrs. Jones. How would you like to make payment today?*
>
> *Staff member: Your charges for the day are $50, Mrs. Jones. We accept major credit cards, personal check, and, of course, cash.*
>
> *Staff member: Your charges for the day are $50, Mrs. Jones. As we told you when you scheduled the appointment, we require the patient's portion of the payment during each visit. How would you like to pay for that? We have several convenient options.*

These are tactful, professional ways for the checkout clerk to carry out the policy and to ensure that appropriate balances are collected at the time of service.

If, for some reason, the patient indicates an inability to make a payment, the clerk should call the billing manager (or, in a smaller practice, the practice manager). The goal is to resolve the situation before the patient leaves. Typically, the clerk who checks out the patient is not authorized to deviate from procedure and will transfer the discussion and decision to the manager. The manager should take the patient to a private room to discuss payment. The element of authority imposed by the billing or practice manager indicates that nonpayment is unacceptable. At the discretion of the manager, the patient may be allowed to leave without paying, but, preferably, with an agreed-upon plan for payment.

For sizeable balances that insurance plans do not pay or for high deductibles that have not been met, the practice manager or designated staff member can help the patient find an acceptable way to pay for the medical care. Educating the patient on what to expect, both medically and financially, increases the likelihood of collecting. Preauthorized credit card payments and in-house time payment plans are suitable methods of collecting payment for services. **Form 5-1** is a sample of a financial agreement for insurance patients who need to pay their bills over time.

The long-range goal is to develop the understanding that arrangements for payments must be made in advance of the encounter. As with most matters related to credit and collection policy, it is essential to be consistent across the patient base. Consistent patterns of collection inform both the staff and the patients that direct patient payment is important. It's your money. Ask for it!

FORM 5-1. SAMPLE FINANCIAL AGREEMENT

FINANCIAL AGREEMENT

Patient: _____

Person responsible for payment: _____

Address: _____

City: _____State: _____Zip: _____

Home phone: _____Business phone: _____Other:_____

Description of services:

Fee for services $_____

Estimate of insurance benefits $_____

Estimate of patient portion $_____

Payment plan options:
❑ I prefer paying 100% of the patient portion of what the insurance does not cover on the first (   ) appointment.

❑ I prefer paying 50% of the patient portion of the first (   ) appointment. The remainder to be paid within 15 days after the insurance has paid their portion.

In the event the account should become delinquent for a period of thirty (30) days, I hereby acknowledge that I will be responsible for all the balance, interest, court costs, and/or attorney fees.

I hereby certify that I have read and received a copy of the foregoing disclosure statement this _____

date of _____, 2_____.

Signature: _____, Responsible Party

CONFIRMING AND GATHERING THE COPAYMENTS

One of the challenges facing medical practices today is making sense of varying insurance and managed care plans and associated payment policies, including the amounts of copays and deductibles for which the patient is responsible. To collect payment from the patient when services are rendered, staff members need to know what each plan calls for, and they should be able to relate that information assertively to the patient at the time of check-out.

Not only does failing to collect payment at time of service hurt the practice initially because of the absence of cash flow, but billing after the fact is also costly. Because it can be difficult to collect a small copayment, the practice may allow such payments to be ignored. Thousands of dollars are involved over the year and the loss of this money directly affects the bottom line by increasing the practice's net collections and net-to-gross charge relationship. To maintain patient payment responsibility:

- maintain an up-to-date reference of the patient's account balance at the check-out station and
- allow different forms of payment, including credit cards, for the unpaid balance.

It is very important to keep a handy reference to each plan's specification in the check-out area. Information about all the plans in which the practice participates should be available. In vertical columns across the page, list each procedure's regular charge, what that plan allows and disallows, and the deductible or copayment for which the patient is responsible.

One way to gather this information is from the plan's representative. An alternative is to review explanations of benefits (EOBs) from each plan. This summary table should be updated periodically so the most current amounts are received. Do not assume that the same deductible or copay exists from year to year. Plans change often, and many times the first thing that changes is the copay amount. Patients change employers as well, so it is wise to get the information and confirm it in several directions. Front office staff members should check the patients' insurance cards. The copay amount is listed on them. This is the best way to check because an insurance company can have a high and low option plan indicating $5 or $10 copays respectively.

With this type of information, the practice's front office personnel will have a way to determine what the patient owes and will be expected to pay before leaving the office. It is essential to ask for payment. Train your staff to handle the requests with ease.

Often, the excuse for not paying the copay or deductible is, "I didn't bring my checkbook." For this reason, most practices accept credit card payment. Except in very poor areas, most adults carry at least one major credit card. Accepting credit cards entails a discounting fee, which is paid to the credit card carrier. However, it allows for immediate payment and makes paying more convenient for the patient.

In some managed care plans, the contract specifically prohibits collecting deductibles and/or copays until the plan has paid. (These are different from the copays required at time of service.) If possible, negotiate this out of the contact. If the contract does have this provision, however, obtain advance authorization as a guarantee on payment when large amounts are at stake. (This payment mechanism is similar to that used by car rental agencies and hotels.) Major credit card companies provide forms for patients to sign in advance. This will authorize credit card charges on receipt of partial insurance payments. Ask the patient what maximum charge limit applies to the card to ensure that an excessive amount will not be charged.

When credit cards are accepted in advance for payments due after treatment, the practice should send a zero-balance statement to the patient when the charge is made to the credit card. The statement should show the amount due after insurance payment and note that this amount was paid by credit card. Sending out a statement showing the payment transaction will minimize the need for patients to call with questions about a payment. **Table 5-1** outlines six principles for collecting the self-pay portion from patients before they leave your practice.

TABLE 5-1. SIX PRINCIPLES FOR COLLECTING THE SELF-PAY PORTION FROM PATIENTS

1. Train your staff about the importance of colleting self-pay amounts.

2. Know which patients are self-pay, and ensure the cashier or exit receptionist handles the collection on exit.

3. Keep a cash fund to make change for $5, $10, and $20 bills. Have a simple system to reconcile and replenish the fund at the end of each day.

4. Encourage credit card payment. Except in very low-income environments, most patients carry a credit card with them.

5. Arrange for automatic credit card charge by using a preauthorized health care form. The patient can authorize charging copays, deductibles, and other charges for all visits during a year. Asking your patient to sign the form on the first visit takes care of the collection hassle for the rest of the year.

6. Enforce self-pay. If a patient refuses to pay as called for under the contract with the carrier, send a bill with a special notice. This will remind the patient of the requirement to pay and indicate that you will notify the HMO if the patient refuses to pay.

RECOGNIZING THE IMPORTANCE OF COPAYMENTS

Copays are an important source of revenue and have a significant financial effect on the medical practice. Collection of copays is a fundamental component of managed care. In general, when copayments are not collected, utilization increases. Insisting on patient payment helps educate patients to seek medical treatment only when they really need it. Also, practices that do not collect copays are violating their contracts with payers who require them.

Although copays are seemingly small amounts, particularly with HMOs, collecting them is important. The typical copay is as low as $3 to $5, or as high as $20 to $25. If you see four patients an hour, a $2 copay amounts to at least $5,000 a year for a specialist and $10,000 yearly for a primary care doctor. To discover the potential effect of copays in your practice, multiply the number of patients you see each day by the average copay, and then multiply that number by the number of days you practice each year. For example:

$$40 \text{ patients per day} \times \$10 = \$400$$
$$\$400 \times 264 \text{ days per year} = \$105,600$$

The best way to collect this money is to get it over the counter when services are provided. The cost of sending out statements for copays is essentially prohibitive and seldom results in collection. Unless there is a large balance, trying to collect small amounts is expensive. Small amounts due are often ignored by the patient. Often, he or she assumes the amount is an error or does not want to be bothered to write a check, mail, or use a stamp for such a small balance.

ESTABLISHING COLLECTION GOALS

A practical way of ensuring payment at the time of service is by setting collection goals. This allows for easy tracking and evaluation of adherence. Recommendations for collection goals are

- 100% of all copays and
- 80% of all other types of balances, including Medicare's 20% if the patient does not have supplemental insurance.

Monitor collection on a regular basis, using daily reports to compare the number of copayments and balance bills collected with the number that should have been paid. **Form 5-2** will help you perform this analysis.

FORM 5-2. COLLECTION SUCCESS ANALYSIS

MONTH OF _____

Day	Total Office Visits	Total Subject to Patient Payments	Total Office Visits with Patient Payment Received	% Payable Visits to Total Office Visits	% PATOS (payment at time of service) to Total Subject to Total Subject to Payment	% Goal
Totals						

Month Summary   Total Office Visits   _____

Total Visits with Payment Due   _____   (__%)

Total Visits with Payment Received   _____   (__%)

Year-To-Date Summary   Total Office Visits   _____

Total Visits with Payment Due   _____   (__%)

Total Visits with Payment Received   _____   (__%)

TABLE 5-2. FRONT OFFICE COLLECTION POLICY EFFECTIVENESS AUDIT

1. Select a sample of patient office visits (between 10 and 30 separate days).

2. Tabulate all of the visits in which patient payments at the time of service were applicable. This should include self-pay patients who should have paid in full or part and patients making copays and deductibles. Exclude visits in which the practice cannot legally accept payment (eg, Medicaid, workers' compensation, and some managed care plans).

3. Count the number of visits in which the patients actually made payments.

4. Divide the number of payments by the number of potential payments to compute the percentage of patients making payments at the time of their visits. The higher the percentage, the more efficient the collection process.

Once policies are established and adherence becomes part of the daily routine of the practice, you can increase the goals for point-of-service collection, which include copays, deductibles and self-pay balances.

Conduct periodic audits to evaluate the effectiveness of the collection policy by analyzing the percentage of the office visits that are actually paid (at least partially) while the patients are being seen. **Table 5-2** describes the typical steps to perform such an audit. The goals of collecting 100% of all appropriate copays and 80% of other patient-responsible balances may be aggressive at first, but they are attainable.

Often, precedents set by other local practices and by previous providers in the same practice have a bearing on the practice's collection policy. In some communities, the standard is to bill a patient's insurance before attempting to collect from the patient. Even if this process is the established mode and is expected by patients in the service area, change may be appropriate and necessary. Today's health care environment demands better fiscal management and compliance with contract provisions.

MAKING THE MOST OF BALANCE BILLING

If the patient fails to make complete payment at the time of service, it will be necessary to implement another method to collect the amount due. We recommend handing patients who do not pay at the time of service an itemized copy of charges before they leave the practice. This not only informs them of their responsibility; it also clearly communicates that payment will be due soon.

After third-party payments have been collected, the remaining outstanding balances will be the responsibility of the patient. **Table 5-3** illustrates the typical scenario.

This adjustment process should be clearly outlined in the contracts with the managed care providers. Therefore, the patient and the practice staff should understand this process from the start. Usually, the final balance will be outstanding at the conclusion of payment by the third-party payer. Balance billing must also be addressed so that the practice receives all monies due.

TABLE 5-3. TYPICAL PATIENT PAY SCENARIO

1. Patient copay is collected.

2. Practice bills for charges associated with visit on HCFA 1500 or electronically through a clearinghouse. (HCFA 1500 is a standard claim form developed by the Health Care Financing Administration.)

3. Insurance or other third party pays a fee-schedule amount (usually less than the billed amount).

4. Payment amount minus billed amount equals adjustment amount or balance due.

5. Patient is billed balance due via a statement.

6. If payment is not received, patient is sent collection letter(s).

7. Patient is phoned about balance and payment setup.

Most insurance companies allow patients to assign benefits directly to the health care provider. This does not require an arrangement between the physician and the third-party payer or insurance company. It is preferable to encourage the patients to assign benefits. Doing so will enhance the likelihood of collection with very little risk to the patient. However, it should be pointed out to the patient that the assignment of benefits directly to the physician does not relieve the patient of responsibility for payment. While it assures the physician of collecting the fees that the insurance company is contractually obligated to pay, the ultimate responsibility is the patient's.

Many practices defer sending patient statements until they have ascertained how much the insurance has paid and therefore how much patients owe. There are different schools of thought pertaining to this matter. Some practices prefer sending bills before insurance has been paid to demonstrate that the patient is ultimately responsible for payment. On the other hand, it may alarm a patient to see a large outstanding balance when insurance has not paid its portion—which is normally the greater amount of the total fee. Also, since many patients realize that insurance has not yet paid, they disregard the bill. Thus, sending bills before receiving insurance payments can be a waste of time and effort and not worth the cost.

The practice therefore must determine the best way to proceed. It is most common to wait to send patient bills until the insurance company has been billed and the resulting residual balance ascertained. If the practice is doing an efficient job of collecting copays and deductibles up front, balance billing will not be as big an issue.

Regardless of when balance billing takes place, at some point the third-party payer will fulfill its financial obligation to the practice. At that point, the practice must aggressively pursue payment from patients. As a part of the practice's overall collection plan, it must have in place a set of protocols to inform patients of the status of their accounts and of the financial and time obligations once third-party payers have fulfilled their financial obligations. A consistent financial policy must clearly outline the practice's requirements for the patient's ultimate payment responsibility. The patient and all staff members need to know what the policy is.

Many times, front office staff members are confused about whether physicians can see and treat certain categories of patients. For example, staff members don't know whether physicians will see the following types of patients:

- patients who haven't made payments on their delinquent accounts for a certain period,
- managed care patients who arrive for appointments without primary care referrals, and

- patients required to make copayment at time of service who have no money, check, or credit card with them.

Obviously, a consistent plan must be followed, with few exceptions. Physicians may desire to see the patients but, because of these policies, simply cannot. This should be handled in a professional and consistent manner.

An inconsistent financial policy can cause considerable frustration and even embarrassment for staff members. Ultimately, monies will be lost if there are inconsistencies in the financial policy. If no such policy exists, for example, physicians will treat most patients, and the practice will not be paid for services it renders.

Practices that send statements on a regular basis (whether before or after third-party payers have remitted their portion) should complete and mail them on a monthly basis. Often, the statements are mailed at the end of the month, so they will arrive early the following month. The hope is that this coincides with the time during which patients pay their other bills. Many practices do cycle billing. This is when the patient accounts are divided into four groups and group one (eg, A-F) statements are sent out week one; group two (G-M) are sent out week two, and so on.

If statements are sent before receipt of insurance reimbursement, a note should clearly indicate the pending insurance payment. If no mention of pending insurance payment is made, patients may pay the balance, creating a credit in their account, or they may be upset because they incorrectly assume that the insurance company has refused payment.

Some practices selectively write off a remaining balance without sending the patient an account statement. This should not be done under any circumstance, unless the balance is so small that it would cost more than the amount of payment to send the statement. The routine writing off of copayments and deductibles is illegal, especially for Medicare patients. Therefore, the practice should always make an effort to collect these balances.

Another aspect of balance billing is application of a finance charge for overdue balances. While this is becoming more prevalent, most medical practices do not apply such charges. In most states, a person must have agreed in writing to pay a finance charge. Moreover, a finance charge often violates provider agreements with insurance companies or other third-party payers. With Medicare, it would be a violation because it would increase the amount a physician collected to more than the allowable fee. This is the case whether the practice is a participating or nonparticipating provider. In addition, finance charges may violate managed care arrangements because most such contracts stipulate the physician cannot collect more than the copayment and deductible from the patient.

Nonetheless, as legal precedents are established and patients begin to accept it, practices should consider applying finance fees to overdue bills. Of course, if they have done an effective job of collecting copayments and deductibles up front (as they should), it would be a moot point.

CONCLUSION

It is crucial for a practice to collect all the money due directly from the patient. Timing is important. Because the typical balance owed by the patient is considerably less than 50% of the total bill, the sooner this balance can be received, the better. Most managed care plans require the collection of copays and deductibles. Generally, they can be collected at any time, though it is preferable to collect them at the time services are rendered. Doing so maximizes cash flow and overall collections as a percent of charges.

Often, practices will have some self-pay patients with little or no insurance coverage. In other cases, specific services may not be covered by insurance. In these instances, the practice should work out a specific payment plan collecting as much as possible up front. Often, this will coincide with the timing of the services. For example, after elective cosmetic surgeries are completed, postoperative services allow a time frame in which to spread out payments. (Note, however, that all elective cosmetic surgeries are paid for up front.) Nonetheless, the practice should have a definitive payment plan for these patients.

In this era of reduced reimbursements and continuing financial pressures, patient payment of balances is ever more important. Whether collection is a legal or contractual obligation should not matter. What is important is that the collection of copays, deductibles, and other patient-responsible payments is good business.

CHAPTER 6

Getting Paid by Insurers

A third party normally pays most of the total professional charges generated by a physician's office. This third party may be an insurer, such as an HMO, a preferred provider organization, or an insurance company with a standard indemnity insurance plan. There are many types of private carriers, including health plans that are owned by or affiliated with such health care facilities as hospitals. The other major third-party payer is the US government, primarily through Medicare or Medicaid. We will examine Medicare's payment processes in Chapter 7.

Physicians may at times be distressed if the cost of services to maintain or enhance a patient's quality of life places that patient under economic stress. Third-party insurers assume the financial risks associated with patient health care and are expected to alleviate economic stress on both patients and providers. As the cost of health care delivery has continued to increase, third-party insurers are under greater pressure to reimburse at acceptable levels.

In the United States, most health care insurance is provided by thousands of employers to employees and dependents. Typically, employers contract with third-party insurers. Usually, a portion of the cost is passed on to employees, with the bulk of the premium being paid by the employer.

Insurance companies do not accept the premise that all claims should be paid as submitted. The health care provider must submit an accurate and timely claim, with sufficient documentation, to receive payment. Often, this requires special approval or preauthorization before health care service is provided.

In many instances, third parties require special billing forms, medical procedure and diagnosis coding, and contractual relationships. As a result, the medical office needs to have a sophisticated credit and collection policy for its patients and must adhere to the policy as closely as possible. In addition, it should have consistent billing methods to accommodate the third-party insurer, ensuring that all information is provided on the claim to ensure reimbursement and to avoid delayed reimbursement.

Frequently, the physician must also know what the insurer considers the appropriate processes and relative values for services being performed. The insurance company must credential the physician, and this often requires the physician's own personal profile, which includes such information as home address, medical school, malpractice carrier information, references, and published works.

SUBMITTING A CLEAN CLAIM

Once a patient encounter is complete, the physician's office is responsible for providing adequate and complete information to enable the third-party insurer to promptly process and pay the claim. A breakdown in the process will delay payment or possibly preclude it.

As a result, the process for submitting a clean claim must be supported by a thorough and fully workable billing process. The process includes the following three phases: preappointment, appointment, and postappointment.

The preappointment phase is often the best time to verify insurance. If the patient has changed insurance carriers, which happens quite often, then the earlier the better for this to be documented in the practice's information system. That way, additional data can be compiled before the appointment or authorization can be obtained from the third-party insurer. There may be a different deductible and copay, as well as specific areas of authorization and verification of coverage.

Four important steps occur during the appointment. First, patient information should again be verified. This entails confirming all demographic information about the patient, so that proper documentation and coding can be completed. (This was discussed in Chapter 5.) Second, the physician has to properly document the services that were performed, and either the physician or the coding assistant must translate that documentation into correct CPT codes. Third, the charge capture process must be completed. This usually entails summarizing all codes for each patient encounter and relating them to the practice's fee schedule. Finally, the time of service payment (as discussed in Chapter 4) is essential during the appointment phase.

After the appointment is completed, several processes must take place. These processes are the focus of this chapter. There are eight major initiatives that must be completed properly:

- prebilling,
- claims transmission,
- payer follow-up,
- payment posting,
- denial management,
- statement generation,
- collections, and
- retrospective and concurrent review.

Prebilling

The first part of the postappointment process, which is part of the overall goal of submitting a clean claim, is prebilling. Prebilling protocols should be encompassed within regular coding reviews, periodic account reviews of payments, insurance changes and collection activities, and a claims edit process. In effect, these areas of maintenance should be addressed as a function of the management of accounts receivable.

These areas are often neglected. There may not be a staff member who is responsible for the process, or time is not allotted for appropriate individuals to complete this analysis. Nonetheless, it must be completed regularly.

The claims edit process is a useful tool. There are software packages being developed that will complete the "claim-scrubbing" process before the actual claim submission. One such software now on the market examines a claim for accurate ICD-9 and CPT linkage prior to claim release. Using such software will verify the legitimacy of the claim prior to its submission.

Claims Transmission

Essentially, there are two ways to process claims. The first is on paper and is mostly a manual process that uses traditional mail. The second, and certainly more preferred, is electronic.

Paper claims submission provides slow turnaround and payment (normally 45 days or more). In some cases, these claims are also reflective of secondary filings where they represent a claim filed with a secondary source of payment (eg, Medigap) or a supplemental payer (eg, a liability carrier). Presently, many paper claims are filed for procedural services in which the operative notes must be matched to the claim and submitted with the claim for reimbursement. This is also true for many surgery services.

Electronic filing is becoming more popular. It can be used for most governmental reimbursement and with large commercial payers. Typically, a clearinghouse processes the claim after it is submitted electronically by the medical practice. This provides the fastest turnaround for payment. Editing and checking behind the claim is required. Ensure that the clearinghouse is submitting all claims that you have contracted to have submitted. Check the report provided by the clearinghouse of those "suspended claims" and determine why they were not sent.

Payer Follow-Up	Constant follow-up with payers is essential. Usually, for electronic filings follow-up should be done within 21 days of filing if no payment has been received. For manual or paper filings, follow-up is needed in 45 days. The practice should obtain a report that summarizes the open items by payer. Automatic rebilling should not be completed until or unless some communication has taken place or the practice has a working knowledge of the account balance and its situation. Of course, the rule is to promptly follow up on claims before they age too much.
Payment Posting	When the EOB is received from the insurance company, it should be processed, and payments should be posted accurately to the payer and patient account. This should be done on a daily basis. Feedback should be given to the physicians and nurses in regard to coverage for certain CPT codes from the EOB. Was the service coded correctly? Could it be coded differently?
Denial Management	Part of follow-up is consistently analyzing claims that have been denied. Denied claims should be summarized by type of payer and analyzed to ascertain why they were denied. This should help avert denial in the future.
Statement Generation	Accurate statement generation should follow the submission of a clean claim. Statements should be sent on a regular basis, at least monthly, to both the patient and the third-party insurance company. Statements should be separated by the insurance balance and the patient's responsibility. As balances are delayed or age, follow up on them and include the follow-up as part of the ongoing record keeping. Follow-up can also include such actions as including dunning messages on statements.
Collections	Collection is a unique feature of the accounts receivable management process. It is examined in detail later in the chapter.

Analyze key accounts receivable reports throughout the postappointment phases. These reports include

- Aging reports
- Days in accounts receivable
- Reports of total denials
- Other pertinent items of information, such as adjustment percentages and write-offs.

Retrospective and Concurrent Review

Figure 6-1 is a flowchart summarizing the typical processes for submitting a clean claim. It illustrates the processes for both manual and electronic filing. Each procedure must be completed for the claim to be paid in a timely and accurate manner. Furthermore, it is important to continuously evaluate these processes to ensure that no breakdowns have occurred. For example, a greater number of denials signals a high likelihood that a malfunction has taken place.

Once the procedures are documented and monitored, specific adherence to the required documentation and form-filing compliance are needed. Often, claims are not accepted because they include incomplete or inaccurate information. **Table 6-1** summarizes items that may stand in the way of the submission of clean claims. If a practice continuously monitors these items to ensure that they are handled appropriately, there will be a greater likelihood of clean claim submission and prompt payment.

DEVELOPING PAYER PROFILES AND ANALYSES

It is not good business practice for a physician to ignore third-party payers. In fact, it is essentially impossible to ignore them, since they make most health care payments. A physician who ignores third parties and places the full burden of paying for services on the patients not only does them a disservice, but also will likely have a very small practice.

As a result, physicians and staff members must be familiar with how third-party reimbursement works and what can be done to obtain the most from these payers. If a direct contract with the third party exists, errors in billing will result in a direct loss to the practice. At the very least, errors will result in payment delay.

The credit manager should be familiar with the various third-party payers and should know their requirements better than the patient does. Emphasis should be placed on third parties that represent the greatest number of patients in the practice.

FIGURE 6-1. CLAIMS PROCESSING FLOWCHART

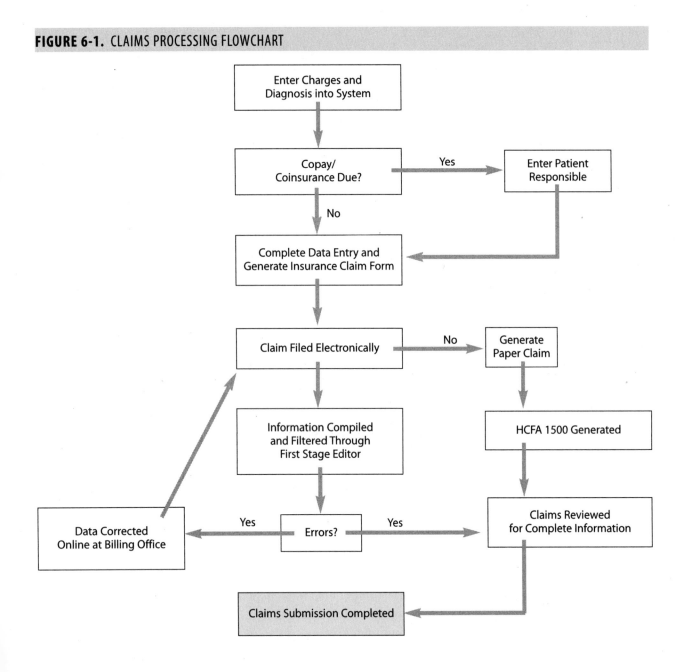

TABLE 6-1. CLEAN CLAIM INTERVENTIONS

The following are common reasons that claims are not clean claims:

Assignment	Accept assignment box checked inappropriately
Authorization	Claim form did not list the mandatory authorization number or referral form is missing.
CPT-4	Invalid CPT-4 code
Codes	Invalid revenue codes printing on a UB82 facility claim. Medicaid emergency code, injury code, resources code, other insurance code and/or Medicare status code invalid or missing. Centers input invalid insurance codes, ie, 999 (unknown).
Contract Number	Subscriber's contract number missing or invalid
Dates	Missing or incorrect dates, such as admission and discharge dates, duplicate dates of service for same procedure code, dates of last menstrual period, first symptom, etc.
Diagnosis	Diagnosis code missing or invalid
Group Number	Missing group number on claim form
ID Number	Physician's provider ID or license number missing on claim form
Incorrect Balance	Incorrect balance printing on claims. Claims involving coordination of benefits have to be manually adjusted to reflect the correct payment received and amount due.
Insurance Info.	Subscriber's name, subscriber's sex, social security number, group and/or plan number missing or invalid. Medicare ID cannot have a space or hyphen between the numeric and alpha character. Names must appear exactly as they appear on the patient's card.
Modifiers	Missing modifier on a procedure that mandates usage of one
Other	Units (quantity) are incorrect and are manually changed or deleted on UB82 claims for Blue Cross facility charges.
Patient Info.	Patient's gender missing or invalid, patient's address invalid, birth date missing, etc
Physician Notes	Procedures that always require documentation are not matched with documentation. Documentation is requested from the appropriate source.
Place	Place of service incorrect **1.** Inpatient **2.** Outpatient **3.** Physician's office
Primary Sponsor	Medicaid recipients who have a primary sponsor must reflect the primary sponsor's name, ID, and type on professional and/or facility claims.
Private Payer Service Code	Private payer service code missing or invalid
Provider	Provider (physician) information missing or incorrect (ie provider ID, license number, etc)
Referral	Referring physician's name and/or ID missing on claim form
Type Number	Type of bill incorrect on facility claims. Type of bill varies according to first time claim, status, coordination of benefits, etc.
Type Service	Type of service listed incorrectly on claim form

Most third-party insurers have specific participation contracts that specify how they agree to reimburse physicians. Thus, it is important to develop a summary or profile of each third-party insurer. Profiles should include each payer's contractual requirements for reimbursement and its procedural protocols. It is virtually impossible to keep up with this information without some type of automated summary. Continually evaluate and update the summary so that it is current. This information will assist both the billing and collection staff. Further, if the summary is up-to-date, it is more likely that claims will be clean.

Although many practices keep this information themselves, commonly payer profiling is best completed by a central processing organization (CPO), such as a management services organization, an independent practice association (IPA), or some other service organization that can maintain data on an up-to-date basis. Regardless of the means by which the information is maintained, each practice should have a complete and thorough update of its payers' profiles, particularly of the most prominent payers. The profiles should be analyzed on a regular basis to ascertain the methodologies, procedures and overall appropriateness of reimbursement. **Forms 6-1** and **6-2** can be used to develop such profiles.

DEALING WITH SLOW INSURANCE PAYERS

Typically, there is a huge variance in the promptness of payments by third-party insurers. Some payers are very responsive and pay within a reasonable time of claim submission. Others seemingly deliberately withhold payment as long as possible. It appears that the "one who barks the loudest" traditionally receives faster payment.

Include the characteristics and reputation for timeliness of payments in the evaluation of each third-party insurer. Then, when you evaluate and negotiate managed care contracts, make sure to consider timeliness. Contact other medical offices or perhaps the state insurance commission to ascertain the reputation of the third-party insurer. Many times, problems can be averted by early knowledge of the third parties' reputation.

In addition, consider adding language to the contract to require the insurance company to pay within a certain number of days from claim submission. Usually, this is in the 30- to 40-day range, with a shorter amount of time for electronic claim filing.

Once the claim has aged, dealing with the slow payer becomes more problematic. The best solution is to constantly monitor accounts so that no payer's balances extend beyond a reasonable period. For example, once an account has reached the 45-day point, the practice should contact the insurance company.

FORM 6-1. PAYER PLAN PROFILES (INCLUDES SPECIFIC MANAGED CARE PLANS)

Payer Plan Name and TPO	Employer	Number of Employees	Copay	Recommended Withhold Percent	Fee Basis	Claims Turn-around Time	Renewal Date Termination Rights	Time Limits on Filing	Hold Harmless Clause?	Hospital Providers	Laboratory Providers	Radiology Providers	Other Ancillary Providers

FORM 6-2. PAYER ORGANIZATION PROFILES (INCLUDES SPECIFIC THIRD-PARTY ORGANIZATIONS)

Payer	Contact/ Phone	Employer	Fee Structure	ID Card Description	Copay	Benefit Exclusions	Hospital	Lab	X-ray	Other	Renewal Date	Referral by Physician Plan (Identified by the Practice)

It is best to have a direct relationship with an account representative from the third party. Such a relationship will not only allow easier access to the insurance company, it will also enable a more responsive series of actions, ultimately resulting in a prompter payment.

If these methods prove to be unsuccessful, get more aggressive. Send statement filings, make telephone calls, and contact the state insurance commissioner. Another way to influence payment is to have patients contact the insurance company directly or express concern to their employer, asking the employer to request payment from the insurance company. When the patient is reminded that the balance due is his or her responsibility, this will accelerate the patient's interest in resolving the matter. **Table 6-2** summarizes ways to bill and collect from slow insurance payers.

Every medical practice should use a series of collection letters to obtain payments on delinquent third-party insurer and patient accounts. Ideally, the computer system should generate these letters automatically. Many systems have this excellent collections tool, but often, practices do not use it appropriately or at all. All staff members who have collections responsibilities should learn to use this automated feature.

When possible, the computer system should also automatically generate statements for accounts on which no payments have been made in the last 60, 90, and 120 days. Occasionally, a balance is delinquent because of miscommunication. Statements provide prompt recognition of this outstanding balance owed to the practice.

TABLE 6-2. SUCCESSFUL WAYS TO BILL AND COLLECT FROM PAYERS

1. Develop expertise by payer.

2. Have systems in place to identify improper, inaccurate and underpaid remittances.

3. Use an automated process to ask for and supply information.

4. Establish performance standards for collectors (number of claims worked per day, dollars collected, aging of accounts, etc). Establish performance-based incentive pay.

5. Require supervisory personnel to follow up on unpaid checks aged over 120 days.

6. Establish a summary feedback-to-charge source.

7. Require (allow) physicians and practice managers to have strategic input and operational influence.

8. Make certain payers know that if they delay payments, they will be aggressively pursued. Speak with a supervisor.

9. Review performance of accounts receivable by provider and payer. Require collectors to monitor this also.

10. Institute and follow a system for addressing unpaid or rejected claims.

IDENTIFYING INCORRECT PAYMENTS

The practice staff is responsible for identifying inaccurate, incorrect, or insufficient payments. It is highly unlikely that the insurance company will ever note such problems.

Most insurance companies are large bureaucracies. They generally follow specific rules and standards and rarely make exceptions. Therefore, the onus is on the practice to find mistakes and aggressively correct them.

Begin by consistently reviewing all EOB forms. Most EOB forms from insurance companies are explicit. They outline not only what is being paid, but also what services have been provided and the amount being paid for each patient. The EOB says what is not covered and why. Specific action needs to be taken to cover this if possible and resubmit the claim immediately. Even if an EOB includes payment that encompasses many patients (as Medicare payments often do), there is sufficient individual information to complete an analysis. A practice must have a standard policy of reviewing EOBs without exception.

Once incorrect payments have been identified, staff members must immediately contact the insurance company. It helps if you have already developed rapport with someone—possibly a customer service representative—at the insurance company. Preferably, your contact is a supervisor. If not, a supervisor should be contacted as needed during disputes.

To determine whether you need to speak with a supervisor, ask the customer service representative whether he or she would be able to solve your problem if they agree with your position. If the answer is "no," find out who the supervisor is and continue the discussion with that individual. If the answer is "yes," determine whether the customer service representative has true authority to resolve the claim at this point or if the supervisor should nonetheless be contacted.

Although it is very rare, some insurance companies require practices to use specific forms for their claims. These companies also create their own procedure codes instead of using CPT™ codes. If such an insurance company represents only a small part of the practices' patient base, the practice may decide to terminate the relationship with the insurance company because of its bureaucracy. Usually, the best option is to segregate these claims and have a particular employee learn the system and work the claims as a separate batch.

It is important to have time standards and sequence for collection activities. The process must move along as rapidly as possible and not get bogged down in the daily activities of the regular billing process. If a mistake has resulted in an underpayment, it is not costing the insurance company anything for resolution to be delayed.

We recommend charting the performance of each payer. This should include the total number of incorrect payments versus the total number of claims and the number of days of follow-up and the time expended to collect correct payment. This simple process will help you monitor insurance companies that consistently submit incorrect payments.

Monitoring the outstanding accounts receivable via a thorough and complete aging schedule will also alert the billing manager about accounts that are problematic. Once a payment has been posted, the only difference that should remain is that between the gross charge and the agreed-on contractual amount. Some contractual agreements require this balance to be written off. Others allow you to bill the patient for the balance. Often, practices do not write off the difference between their gross and net charges when payments are received. This makes it hard to ascertain whether an amount left on an account is a result of underpayment. Thus, it is very important to write off these balances at the time of receipt of payment if this is the practice's policy.

AUTOMATING REQUESTS FOR INFORMATION FROM THE PROVIDER

A practice must be able to communicate using automated, interactive processes in order to substantiate its services. Instantaneous communication prevents time lost in the mail system, lost paper, and telephone tag. More and more insurance companies are capable of processing electronically submitted claims. **Table 6-3** shows the advantages of electronic submission.

TABLE 6-3. ADVANTAGES OF ELECTRONIC CLAIMS SUBMISSION

1. Faster payment

2. Quicker error detection

3. Reduced mailing costs

4. Reduced clerical labor

5. Immediate claim payment or denial response

6. Greater integrity provided to the whole billing process

7. Overall significant money savings for the practice

There are many interactive systems currently available and being developed both by private and hospital-based companies that will assist medical practice providers. The Internet and other e-business mechanisms will be invaluable in the future. Practices that are proactive in learning about what is available in terms of the Internet and other means of electronic communication will likely progress the fastest and have the best operating results.

Commonly, electronic claims are now filed through a clearinghouse, which charges a fee. A practice should evaluate the total cost of electronic submission, including the cost of equipment and these access fees. Most practices have concluded that the advantages far outweigh the additional costs.

Many Web sites are directed to both physicians and patients. These health resource sites provide a variety of services, including pharmacy, personal medical records, in-home heart monitoring, and specialists to answer questions. Physicians can also tap into practice management and other services that help run a practice, including interactive communications for claims submission. Personalization is key to these sites. The health content is encoded, indexed, and filtered. In the future, sites will link patients to their physicians.

Some companies are offering free Web sites to physicians. These sites allow the physicians to access data they need. The next opportunity will be on-line interaction with patients and third-party providers.

INSTITUTING A FOLLOW-UP SYSTEM FOR UNPAID OR REJECTED CLAIMS

Most practices are not receiving all the third-party reimbursements to which they are entitled. For example, a physician group submits 100 insurance claims. Of those, 10 are returned with denial of benefits; 5 are paid at a lower code and then filed; and another 3 are completely unacknowledged. A well-trained billing manager follows up on each claim with a telephone call. The average call will last from 30 minutes to 1 hour. Over a month this could encompass the better part of an entire week of the billing manager or clerk's time.

At the end of the next month, additional rejected claims arrive. Some of the claims from the previous month are still outstanding and subject to further analysis. The onus is on the billing department to follow up on these denied claims.

The first step in reducing rejected or denied claims is an efficient patient-intake system. This will significantly reduce the number of claim denials and rejections. This process entails the full continuum of services all the way from the front desk to billing. We examined this earlier in the book; suffice it to say that without an efficient process, the number of claim denials will grow exponentially.

No degree of proficiency in patient intake will eliminate claim denials and rejections. Most practices work the oldest claims first. In some cases, this is not the best approach. Newer denials and rejections are fresher in the minds of staff members, and working them first typically results in quick resolution. It is easier to capture missing information and correct inaccuracies on newer claims, so it takes less time to resubmit the claim with corrective actions, and the return on investment is better.

Strive to be as current as possible with claim resubmissions. Older denied claims, particularly those that are problematic, should not be neglected. The goal should be to resubmit every claim only once to obtain appropriate reimbursement. Any deferral of payment from an originally filed claim is costly to the practice, if for no other reason than the time involved in collecting the cash.

Patterns should be observed in the resubmission process and in supposedly erroneous or incompletely collected information. Such problems could be caused by any member of the billing collection function, including the physicians themselves. Document the reasons for the denials and share this information with the physicians and the staff members. Once the reasons for a denial have been determined, staff members should be educated to avoid further errors.

The billing manager has the main responsibility for following up on denied claims. If the billing manager does not do the actual work, he or she should continuously monitor the progress of staff members who are working denied claims. Dealing with denied claims requires extra analysis and work, and most people will procrastinate instead of addressing them. It is the job of the billing manager to ensure that denied claims are handled on a regular basis. Good strategies include monitoring the number of denied claims and setting goals for the percentage of claims to be filed correctly. Appropriate employee incentives should be developed, possibly with additional compensation once certain percentage thresholds are met. Conversely, when the percentage of claim denials increase, corrective action or withholding incentive pay may need to be considered.

Another key is the availability and use of monthly reports. If all appropriate monthly reports are completed, there will be information on the number of denied claims. The significance of an unpaid claim in an aging report is the most difficult to interpret, because there is no overt message to indicate a problem. Unpaid claims are typically identified when they age more. To discover this promptly, the billing manager must regularly run aging analyses, examine them closely, and then act on the results.

Addressing a rejected claim is perhaps the billing manager's highest priority. A rejected claim means that professional fees will never be paid unless action is taken. Therefore, in a manner of speaking, these are a higher priority than current claims that may be paid without a problem. Additionally, denial may be a symptom of a larger billing problem that will cause other claims to be denied. If left unattended, the situation could threaten the financial well-being of the practice.

The billing manager should always be thinking of the implications of denied claims, not only as they relate to retrieving those monies, but also in terms of possible trends for future outstanding claims. Implications involving other claims must be addressed immediately. There may be a software or filing procedure problem, or denial may be due to relatively minor errors that may not directly relate to the requested monies.

APPEALING DENIED CLAIMS

Faced with the prospect of wasting valuable staff time on aging claims, a practice will often begin sending statements to patients, hoping that they will make payment. While it is likely that the patient will not pay, he or she may assist in addressing the insurance company.

Too many physicians ignore the single most effective action to secure full payment of denied medical claims—filing an appeal. The reason is that many physicians and billing managers do not know how to file an appeal. Others assume they will not be successful because they are unsure which regulatory guidelines to cite in their favor.

Using Software

Several good software packages aid in the practice for filing appeals. The better ones provide templates for several different appeal letters that cover the most common claim denial reasons. The system automatically provides case law and state statutes to support particular reconsideration. The cost of such software packages is typically reasonable. The prices at the time of this book's publication ranged from a minimum of $500 to as much as $2,000.

To generate an appeal letter, the following information should be entered in the software program: patient information, insurance account, attending physician(s), medical codes, original claim submission dates, and other related data. Then appropriate regulations or legal precedence are cited from the software databases. They could include:

- verification of insurance coverage, including automated on-screen legal forms for benefits verification and assignment;
- local and federal law regarding coverage exclusion, including

preexisting, maternity, newborn, violent crime, and substance abuse
denials;

- state law and medical necessity and utilization review procedures,
  including special rulings on cancer and transplant-related procedures;
- COBRA and ERISA coverage termination legislation; and
- time reprocessing and late payment interest regulations for each state.

Additional software support includes a database of government contact
information for each state, including the insurance commission and
Medicaid offices. In addition, integrated Internet links provide access to
on-line resources such as state legislative databases and national health
care organizations.

Therefore, it is more appropriate to file an appeal using this software
than to rely on a manual system of appeal letters or asking patients to
pursue payment. Patients may have a different definition of medical
necessity or other pertinent language than the practice does, and they may
blame the practice for the making a mistake. A sample claims appeal letter
is shown in **Figure 6-2.**

The Appeals Process

The actual appeals process is fairly well defined by managed care
organizations. Providers and beneficiaries may submit appeals of decisions
regarding treatment and reimbursement. All managed care organizations
have a standard appeal process. If an appeal is necessary, it should be
made in writing, outlining the essential course of action. There are
typically several levels of appeal:

- Urgent review,
- Level 1 appeal,
- Level 2 appeal, and
- Level 3 appeal.

Urgent Review.

If authorization is denied for treatment or post-treatment, a provider
may request immediate phone consultation with the managed care
organization's professional reviewer. Professional reviewers include
psychiatrists, psychologists, and physicians. Only physicians may request
urgent reviews for medical services. Each third-party payer has a specific
protocol of how the appeal is to proceed. However, the appeals process
is generally as follows.

Level 1 Appeal.

Generally, the first appeal is made to the reviewer or clerk who initially

FIGURE 6-2. SAMPLE CLAIM APPEAL LETTER

To: _____

ATTN: PROVIDER APPEALS DEPT.
Address
City, State, Zip

Re:

Insured/Plan Member: _____

ID Number: _____

Group #: _____

Patient Name: _____

Claim #: _____

We are appealing your decision and request reconsideration of the attached claim which
you denied on _____.
We feel these charges should be allowed for the following reason(s):

_____

_____

_____

_____

Thank you for reviewing this claim. Please call if you have any questions at _____.

Sincerely,

rejected or disallowed the claim. This appeal involves a review of the records and claims submitted. The reviewer will probably request the clinical case record from the provider and conduct an additional assessment. The practice should request a quick determination, perhaps as short as 24 hours. It should be pointed out that during this process, the provider is at risk for no authorization of payment of services. An adverse determination at this level entitles the appellant to a Level 2 review.

Level 2 Appeal.

This is usually an appeal to a physician and/or medical director at the managed care organization. It involves a review of the medical records and claims, as well as any additional information supplied by the provider. Some cases will entail a telephone discussion with the provider. Most managed care organizations use a licensed, board-certified physician or licensed nurse, as applicable. An adverse determination at this level entitles the appellant to a Level 3 appeal.

Level 3 Appeal.

This review is commonly conducted by a board or committee composed of providers specializing in the treatment in question. The board reviews all events that have transpired up to that point, as well as relevant documentation and any other information from the parties. In some cases, the board may meet with a provider to hear the facts and to ask questions. This is highly recommended from the provider's standpoint. The review board usually meets weekly.

An adverse determination at this level is frequently considered the final decision unless the third-party payer and the medical practice have contractually agreed to arbitration or the plan is subject to a self-insured employer that provides an additional level of appeal.

Other Stages.

If arbitration is a part of the managed care contract, it will be completed by a designated third party. The arbitrator's decision is typically final and binding. Employers that are self-insured and have hired a third party to administer their insurance plans may require an additional level of appeal. Since self-insured companies effectively make their own rules (within statute restrictions), they can more easily grant exceptions or overrule the insurance administrator. They may also be willing to grant an administrative exemption in support of an employee in good standing. From the provider's standpoint, this is acceptable and preferred in order to obtain the ultimate goal, which is payment for services provided.

Whether the appeal process is made via a software program or administered within the practice or as a part of a defined appeals process, it should be completed in a prompt and orderly manner. As with claim denials and rejections, the burden is on the physician for the loss of reimbursement and working capital to support day-to-day operations. Since the claim will not be paid, in part or full, until the appeals process is completed, timing is of the essence.

There is a right and wrong way to submit an appeal. The wrong way is to resubmit a claim without explaining why it should be reconsidered for payment. The right way is to use a format, as outlined in Figure 6-2, or a more sophisticated software program. Attach the original EOB to the appeal letter. No matter which method is used, the practice should learn from the appeal process.

FILING GRIEVANCES WITH THE STATE INSURANCE COMMISSION

Each state has a regulatory body that oversees the insurance industry. Like most governmental agencies, the insurance commission is intended to be a fair and impartial body that serves the public. Therefore, it should be interested in unfair or potentially unlawful actions by the insurance companies.

When a medical practice believes it is a victim of unfair treatment by an insurance company, it has the right to submit a grievance to the insurance commission. The insurance commission is obligated to investigate the matter and possibly require the insurance company to respond and defend itself. Insurance companies are cognizant of this right. Therefore, leverage is available to the medical practice.

Like most things, filing a grievance takes time and effort. Generally, it is best to consider filing a grievance only in the case of consistent and/or significant problems in which the ramifications of lower reimbursement are great. The practice should pick its battles with insurance companies and not be overly concerned about minor issues.

The appropriate time to file a grievance is for less than appropriate reimbursement, delays in payment, and other perceived inappropriate actions on the part of the insurance company. Contact the state's insurance commission to ascertain the requirements and protocols for filing the grievance.

CONCLUSION

The process of collecting what is rightly due the medical practice from the third-party insurance company or managed care organization involves appropriately implementing all of the procedural processes into billing and collections system functioning. Follow-up and analysis must be regularly executed. Review of aging reports and performance evaluation reports should also be completed on a regular basis.

Dealing with insurance companies can be challenging. They are large and bureaucratic and may try to wield their power and prestige over the relatively small medical practice. They are often difficult to contact, and it is difficult to find a single individual who has the answers to the medical practice's questions. Nevertheless, the medical practice should be consistent and persistent to ensure that matters are resolved.

Some companies are unresponsive to claim inquiries, or take an unreasonably long time to process a claim or forward a payment. If a company is particularly unresponsive, filing a complaint with the state's insurance commission is appropriate. Generally, however, the most effective tactic for dealing with an unresponsive insurer is to involve the patient. This is especially effective if the practice has helped the patient understand that he or she has the ultimate responsibility for payment.

The practice manager or billing manager should routinely review management reports that relate to insurance collection. Reports that are helpful include revenue generated, number of procedures, revenue by insurance company, aging analysis by insurance company, net receipts, contractual adjustments and write-offs, and claim denial rates. Practices that analyze their reports have a much better handle on the situation, and this ultimately results in a more successful collection effort.

It is easy for the process to get out of control. A defined, well-organized and assertive effort that is consistent in its daily approach, follows all policies, and allows few exceptions is essential. If the practice follows these protocols, it will likely be successful in dealing with third-party insurance companies.

CHAPTER 7

Getting Paid by Medicare

To ensure correct remittance by Medicare, staff members must have a working knowledge of Medicare's guidelines for reimbursement. These guidelines are related not only to commensurate coding but to facilitate the administrative process of claims review and payment. Medicare claims must be prepared carefully within the parameters allowed by Medicare to avoid incorrect billing of procedures, which can constitute fraud in the eyes of the government. Thus, it is important to follow the guidelines set forth by HCFA to prepare a clean claim for which payment is remitted in a timely fashion.

KNOW WHAT WILL AND WILL NOT BE PAID

Create a reference chart that shows Medicare covered services similar to the one in **Table 7-1**. This is a good way to ensure that staff members are educated about the breadth of services covered by Medicare. Additionally, the chart will help prevent line item charging for incurred services that are not covered. Patients should be informed up front that fees for procedures not covered by Medicare will be collected at the time of service or filed with a secondary insurer.

KEEP UP WITH POLICY CHANGES

Each year Medicare publishes changes to fees and the allowable procedures in the Federal Register. For example, in 1999, Medicare issued the following change regarding the multiprocedural discount:

TABLE 7-1. SAMPLE MEDICARE COVERED SERVICES CHART

Medicare Services	Coverage
• Medical Expenses: Physician's services; inpatient and outpatient medical and surgical services and supplies; physical, occupational and speech therapy; diagnostic tests and durable medical equipment. Durable medical equipment (DME) includes wheelchairs, walkers, hospital beds, oxygen, etc.	Coverage*
• Clinical Laboratory Services: Blood tests, urinalysis, and more.	Coverage
• Home Health Care: Intermittent skilled care, home health aide services, DME and supplies, and other services.	Coverage
• Outpatient Hospital Services: Services for the diagnosis or treatment of an illness or injury.	Coverage
• Blood: As an outpatient, or as part of a Part B covered service.	Coverage
• X-rays; speech language pathology services; artificial limbs and eyes; arm, leg, back, neck braces; kidney dialysis and kidney transplants • Under limited circumstances, heart, lung, and liver transplants in a Medicare-approved facility • Limited outpatient drugs • Emergency care • Limited chiropractic care • Medical supplies such as ostomy bags, surgical dressings, splints, and casts • Breast prostheses (following a mastectomy) • Ambulance services (limited).	Limited Coverage
Preventive Services: • Screening mammogram • Pap smear, pelvic examination (includes breast exam) • Colorectal cancer screening • Fecal occult blood test • Flexible sigmoidoscopy • Colonoscopy • Barium enema • Diabetes monitoring • Bone mass measurements • Vaccinations: Flu shot, pneumococcal vaccination, Hepatitis B vaccination.	Limited Coverage

*These are covered if they are deemed "medically necessary."

We are replacing the current policy that systematically reduces the practice expense related value units (RVUs) by 50 percent for certain services with a policy that will generally identify two levels of practice expense RVUs—facility and nonfacility—for each procedure code. The higher nonfacility practice expense RVUs will be used for services performed in a physician's office and for services furnished to a patient in the patient's home, or facility or institution other than a hospital, skilled nursing facility (SNF) or ambulatory surgical center (ASC). The lower facility practice expense RVUs will be used for services furnished to hospital, SNF and ASC patients. <u>Note:</u> If a physician performs a procedure at an ASC that is not on the ASC list, use the higher non-facility practice expense RVU.[1]

Additionally, Medicare changed its policy on screening mammograms, Pap smear interpretations, bone density studies, EKG bundling, and anesthesia conversion factors.

After you have ensured that you are billing for items that are covered services and that the coding is accurate, you must have an ongoing awareness of the practice's reimbursement levels. Medicare sends out a monthly bulletin to providers that updates the medical practice concerning coverage issues. This should be read religiously and the information given to physicians and staff members. As a practice manager or other manager, you should calculate a current Medicare fee schedule for your practice, rather than compiling one based on remittance. The formula for calculating the fee schedule is as follows:[2]

Payment = ([RVU Work × GPCI* work] + [RVU practice expense × GPCI] + [RVU malpractice × GPCI malpractice]) × CF

*GPCI = geographic practice cost indices

More information on calculating a fee schedule can be found on the American Medical Association website (http://www.ama-assn.org) under Coding and Medical Information Systems in the RBRVS section or on the HCFA web page (http://www.hcfa.gov).

SUBMIT A CLEAN CLAIM

The 1997 Documentation Guidelines for Evaluation and Management Services published by HCFA and available in print or electronic form provide a systematic listing of the requirements for accurate evaluation and management coding under Medicare.[3] Each provider should have these guidelines readily available, and each billing office should use them to determine claim viability.

In addition, Medicare provides an instruction form for the use of the HCFA 1500, which is the insurance claim form required by Medicare. If you have not read this document, you should. It is available from HCFA in paper and electronic formats. It helps ensure that the claims filed by your practice will never be rejected because of an administrative error.

A clean claim usually consists of the following:

- All fields on the HCFA 1500 are filled, where appropriate.
- All ICD-9 codes are accurately derived.
- All CPT codes represent services rendered that have been adequately documented.
- Services that are included on the HCFA 1500 with a charge are Medicare covered services.

If a claim is returned unpaid, there should be an appeals process in place for the review and investigation of the Remittance Advice from Medicare. Once review and investigation have taken place, if a refile is allowed, file another claim as soon as possible.

USE MEDICARE ELECTRONIC DATA INTERCHANGE (EDI)

Using the Medicare EDI for claims submission and remittance is a necessary first step in accurate and timely claims filing. Advantages include:

- free electronic billing software and support for Medicare claims submission;
- cost-effective electronic transactions that reduce the possibility of error;
- lower administrative, postage, and handling costs than associated with paper claim submissions;
- online receipt and acknowledgement;
- claim status and eligibility information in 24 hours or less;
- electronic remittances sent to a provider-preferred location;
- standardized electronic claims submission and coordination-of-benefits (COB) exchange and remittance receipt, which reduce system costs;
- standardized formats that reduce administrative costs (one format meets all current billing requirements and is accepted by all Medicare contractors as well as many third party billers);
- faster payment on electronic claims (13 days, as compared with 27 days for paper claims); and
- electronic funds transfer (EFT), with accounts receivable in the provider's bank, drawing interest, in two working days (paper checks can take as long as a week to process).[4]

Utilizing EDI and the available error reports allow for a faster arrival at a payable claim. Use this service to its full advantage. It saves time and money.

PAY ATTENTION TO FRAUD: COMPLIANCE SHOULD BE PART OF EVERYDAY BILLING PRACTICES

The prosecution of health care fraud is at an all-time high. Recent legislation has expanded investigators' reach and has increased their power to impose stiff penalties. Investigation and prosecution of health care fraud is a top priority for the Justice Department. This has resulted in an increase in compliance plan development and continuing education in the area of coding.

Physicians are finding themselves increasingly vulnerable. Under the Health Insurance Portability and Accountability Act (HIPAA), physicians may be liable for false claims regardless of whether there was intent to defraud. Moreover, upcoding—using an inaccurate code that would result in a higher payment—is now viewed as a false claim. Because keeping up with changes in evaluation and management codes is extremely difficult, many physicians regularly and unknowingly commit fraud. Several organizations that have been active in providing physicians with compliance guidance are the American College of Cardiology, American College of Surgeons, American Society of Internal Medicine, American College of Physicians, and American Academy of Family Physicians. The American Medical Association and MGMA publish compliance guidelines.

Compliance is part of a process that starts with claim development and submission, with admission and registration, and continues through patient care, coding, and billing. Because fraud can occur in so many ways, ongoing education for all staff members and physicians is essential.

CONCLUSION

Getting paid by Medicare is probably easier than getting paid by most third-party payers, simply because Medicare publishes its rules. All of the guidelines are readily available in electronic and hard copy formats. In addition, continuing education is available on a consulting basis and in seminar format. If you can set up your billing and collections system to accurately file Medicare claims and use this as your benchmark, you will likely file correct claims with commercial payers.

Medicare may provide the lowest reimbursement per procedure for your practice. Nonetheless, use the calculation provided earlier to determine expected reimbursement. If reimbursement falls outside of the expected range, it is your right to bring this to the third-party payer's attention—and you should.

Endnotes

1. Health Care Financing Administration. *Summary of Medicine Physician Fee Schedule Database Changes for 1999.* Baltimore, Md: Health Care Financing Administration; 1999.

2. Health Care Financing Administration. Rules and regulations. *Federal Register,* Baltimore, Md: Health Care Financing Administration; Nov. 2, 1999:64 (No. 211).

3. Health Care Financing Administration. *The 1997 Documentation Guidelines for Evaluation and Management Service.* Baltimore, Md: Health Care Financing Administration; 1999.

4. Health Care Financing Administration. Advantages to using EDI. Available at: http://www.hcfa.gov.

CHAPTER 8

Managing Parallel Payment Systems

The most difficult aspect of managing a billing and collections system is coordinating parallel payment systems. Parallel payment systems are simply those that require a practice to manage both the fee-for-service and the managed or capitated patient.

Whom do I bill, where, and when? The answer to these questions is often fraught with difficulties. Most standard commercial payers accept claim submission via a HCFA 1500, the standard Medicare claim form, and reimburse based on a set fee schedule. However, there are various and sundry hybrids of the standard commercial payer, such as the third-party administrator (TPA), independent practice association (IPA), and provider-sponsored organization (PHO). There are also variations of commercial payer products, such as the HMO product and the capitated contract. Traditionally, there are only two options regarding payment systems:

- Fee-for-service (payment for services rendered at an established rate)
- Managed/capitation (a capped fee for the provision of a set volume of services, which could include carve-out payments for a specialist).

MANAGE ON THE FRONT END

Create a tool, such as the one in **Table 8-1,** for use by the front office staff. It will give staff members the opportunity to assist with the management of payment systems before a claim has been filed. Suggest that staff members refer to the tool at each encounter to be sure that they understand the parameters of the patient's guarantor information.

TABLE 8-1. SAMPLE FRONT OFFICE MANAGED CARE MATRIX

MCO	Copay Deductible/ Other	POS Collection	MD Participation	Preauthorization Requirements	Participating Facilities	Notes
Blue Choice	$10	$10	All	MRI Ultrasound Surgical	St Johns	CAP–**DO NOT BILL FEES–REFFERAL NUMBER REQUIRED FOR VISIT**
PruCare	80/20	20% of encounter total fees	Smith Jones Wilson	MRI Ultrasound Surgical Labor and delivery	St Johns University Hospital	Be sure to copy card– new as of 1/1/00
Cigna	$12	$12	Smith Jones Wilson (NOT Chin)	All radiology Surgical Labor and delivery	St Johns University Hospital Baptist	**REFERRAL NUMBER REQUIRED FOR VISIT**
Create a chart that leaves you room for additions and deletions. Update as you find any new information about a participating payer.						

TABLE 8-2. SAMPLE BACK OFFICE MANAGED CARE REFERENCE MATRIX

MCO	Copay Deductible/ Other	POS Collection	MD Participation	Preauthorization Requirements	Participating Facilities	Front Office Notes	Back Office Notes/Comm on Adjustment
Blue Choice	$10	$10	All	MRI Ultrasound Surgical	St Johns	CAP–**DO NOT BILL FEES–REFFERAL NUMBER REQUIRED FOR VISIT**	Multi-procedural w/o MRI on same claim
PruCare	80/20	20% of encounter total fees	Smith Jones Wilson	MRI Ultrasound Surgical Labor and delivery	St Johns University Hospital	Be sure to copy card– new as of 1/1/00	Second assist w/o provider # Watch for global period cutoff
Cigna	$12	$12	Smith Jones Wilson (NOT Chin)	All radiology Surgical Labor and delivery	St Johns University Hospital Baptist	**REFERRAL NUMBER REQUIRED FOR VISIT**	29909 is discounted below the fee schedule–REFILE with documentation
Create a chart that leaves you room for additions and deletions. Update as you find any new information about a participating payer.							

MANAGE ON THE BACK END

Update the form you created for front office staff members for use by the billing and collections staff. The new form should include all information relevant to the paying history and protocols of the payers. This will make the appeals process much easier for staff members. Have the billing and collections staff meet each week to update the tool. Discussion of the week's claim interactions will be a learning experience. **Table 8-2** is an example of the back office tool.

CAPITATION: VERIFYING COVERAGE AND MONITORING UTILIZATION

Most practices are accustomed to creating an itemized bill for their services. In a capitated environment, the practice may only collect a copay. Unlike its fee-for-service counterpart, the capitated patient has a managed care plan that is based on prepayment for services rather than prospective payment. In such a capitated environment, it is essential that coverage is verified and that accurate copays are collected.

A capitated patient's plan typically pays a flat or capitated fee to the provider, regardless of whether the patient is ever seen. In the same way, the fee paid only covers a certain allowance of procedures such as office visits. The practice must provide this information to the payer for utilization purposes, rather than for the calculation of an allowable or a patient responsibility balance.

There are many variables that must be considered when managing a capitated patient in the practice environment. For example, some prepaid plans require that the patient have authorization prior to a referral and others do not. The understanding of the complex requirements of the capitated patient often require unique training of front office and clinical staff members.

Fewer than half (46.1%) of all payments made by HMOs to primary care physicians are under capitation arrangements. Fee-for-service reimbursements follow at 41.4%. About 9% of payments are fee-for-service plus a withhold. Capitation among specialists is much lower—payments to fewer than one in five specialists were capitated in 1997.[1] Therefore, capitation is probably a small portion of your billing and collections process. Nonetheless, the management of capitation within the practice can be difficult.

Be careful about penalization for overutilization. Penalties are often taken out of withhold money prior to distribution. Yet, despite this trend, more than 75% of HMOs that paid physicians under capitated arrangements did not penalize physicians for such practices as overutilization and excessive referrals. Of the HMOs that reimburse physicians through capitation:

- only one in five penalizes physicians for overutilization of hospitals,
- slightly more than 11% penalize physicians for a violation of prescribing policies, and
- 13% penalize physicians for excessive specialty referrals.[2]

BILLING FOR FEE-FOR-SERVICE CARVE-OUTS

Fee-for-service carve-outs traditionally are involved in contracts where a provider has negotiated a lesser rate for average evaluation and management services and a higher rate for a specific volume of specialty procedures. Usually there are only a few scenarios for carve-outs:

- *Discounted fee-for-service.* The specialty group negotiates a set of rates lower than billed charges. This makes sense for low-volume, very unpredictable courses of treatment with high complication rates. A carve-out can also be a capitated per-member-per-month payment that provides for certain CPT codes as "carved out" and a prenegotiated fee paid in addition to the capitated amount. For example, immunizations and well-woman checkups are frequently "carved out".
- *Case rates.* The specialty provider is paid a flat fee for specific procedures and/or diagnoses for which the group provides special expertise, regardless of volume of services delivered. This is useful for low- and medium-volume and, usually, high-cost procedures in which the specialty group can accurately project cost and utilization.
- *Capitation.* The specialty group receives a flat per-member-per-month payment for a defined patient population. This makes sense for specialties with high-volume, predictable utilization patterns, costs and complication rates.[3]

The carve-out theory of specialty services is behind specialty hospitals such as burn centers, cardiology centers, children's hospitals, and cancer centers. The theory is that the unique expertise, specialized equipment, and higher patient volume will make it possible to deliver better patient outcomes and lower cost than at all-purpose medical facilities. In the past, carve-outs have occurred in the areas of mental health and drug treatment.

Regardless of the form of carve-out, it is another possible nuance in billing and collections management. Ensure that physicians and staff members understand the uniqueness of any carve-out arrangement. More than any other risk arrangement, a carve-out shifts the management burden to the practice.

CONCLUSION

Parallel payment systems can be easily managed with the correct tools. The process begins with a thorough understanding of the practice's managed care contracts, their requirements, and their corresponding fees. This information can then be translated into a usable tool for the entire staff.

Once the participation process has begun, more information can be gathered about the precertification process, the claims payment history, over- and underpayments, adjustments, and so on. All of this becomes valuable information in the management of the system.

If the protocols and tools are in place, management of parallel payment systems is integrated into the overall management of the practice. This is where you want it. You do not want to have a separate system to manage.

The final key to management of the payment systems is ongoing evolution of the tools and protocols. Use the tools and the information they provide to update practice policies and procedures. Make sure that the system is not static—it should evolve as practice evolves.

Endnotes

1. HCIA-Sachs. *Market Profiles for Medicare Risk Contracting.* Baltimore, Md: HCIA-Sachs, 19P98. Item no. MP 2007.

2. Becton, Dickinson and Company, *Report on Physicians in Managed Care.* Franklin Lakes, NJ: Becton, Dickinson and Company, 1997.

3. Soroka L. Specialty carve-outs: Shifting the risk to medical specialty groups. Available at http://www.aispub.com/ManagedCareAdvisor.html. Accessed August 2, 2000.

Benchmarking of Accounts Receivable

1999 Performance and Practices of Successful Medical Groups. Englewood, Colo: Medical Group Management Association; 1999. To order, call: 877-ASK-MGMA (877-275-6462). Online catalog available at http://www.mgma.com.

Ambulatory Surgery Management Society Survey: 1999 Report Based on 1998 Data Benchmarking: Your Practice's Key to Success. Englewood, Colo: Medical Group Management Association; 1999. To order, call: 877-ASK-MGMA (877-275-6462). Online catalog available at http://www.mgma.com.

Cost Survey for the Administrators in Oncology Hematology Assembly: 1999 Report Based on 1998 Data. Englewood, Colo: Medical Group Management Association; 1999. To order, call: 877-ASK-MGMA (877-275-6462). Online catalog available at http://www.mgma.com.

Cost Survey for the Anesthesia Administration Assembly: 1999 Report Based on 1998 Data. Englewood, Colo: Medical Group Management Association; 1999. To order, call: 877-ASK-MGMA (877-275-6462). Online catalog available at http://www.mgma.com.

Cost Survey for the Cardiovascular Thoracic Surgery and Cardiology Assembly: 1999 Report Based on 1998 Data. Medical Group Management Association; 1999. To order, call: 877-ASK-MGMA (877-275-6462). Online catalog available at http://www.mgma.com.

Cost Survey for the Pathology Management Assembly: 1999 Report Based on 1998 Data Cost Survey: 1999 Report Based on 1998 Data. Englewood, Colo: Medical Group Management Association; 1999. To order, call: 877-ASK-MGMA (877-275-6462). Online catalog available at http://www.mgma.com.

Essentials of Benchmarking. Englewood, Colo: Medical Group Management Association; 1999. To order, call: 877-ASK-MGMA (877-275-6462). Online catalog available at http://www.mgma.com.

Benchmarking of Fees

National Fee Analyzer. Item No. 2499, ISBN 1-56337-366-1. Salt Lake City,
Utah: Medicode, Inc; 2000. To order, call 800-999-4600. For more
information, access the Medicode Website at http://www.medicode.com.